Compliments of Canada - Dr
Mark Frost Canada - Dr
P. Clause

Osteoporosis

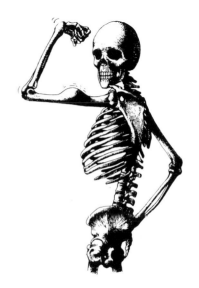

Osteo

porosis

JOHN A. KANIS MD

World Health Organization Collaborating Centre
for Metabolic Bone Disease

Professor in Human Metabolism and Clinical Biochemistry,
Department of Human Metabolism and Clinical Biochemistry,
University of Sheffield Medical School, England

b

Blackwell
Science

I would like to dedicate this book to:
my wife, Monique Benéton and my children:
Lisa, Emma, Sarah, Roobarb and Natalie

© 1994 by
Blackwell Science Ltd
Editorial Offices:
Osney Mead, Oxford OX2 0EL
25 John Street, London WC1N 2BL
23 Ainslie Place, Edinburgh EH3 6AJ
238 Main Street, Cambridge
  Massachusetts 02142, USA
54 University Street, Carlton
  Victoria 3053, Australia

Other Editorial Offices:
Arnette Blackwell SA
1, rue de Lille
75007 Paris
France

Blackwell Wissenschafts-Verlag GmbH
Kurfürstendamm 57
10707 Berlin
Germany

Blackwell MZV
Feldgasse 13
A-1238 Wien
Austria

First published 1994

Set by Setrite Typesetters Ltd,
Hong Kong
Printed in Great Britain
at the Alden Press Limited,
Oxford and Northampton
Bound by Hartnolls Ltd,
Bodmin, Cornwall

DISTRIBUTORS

Marston Book Services Ltd
PO Box 87
Oxford OX2 0DT
(Orders: Tel: 0865 791155
       Fax: 0865 791927
       Telex: 837515)

USA
Blackwell Science, Inc.
238 Main Street
Cambridge, MA 02142
(Orders: Tel: 800 759-6102
         617 876-7000)

Canada
Times Mirror Professional
Publishing, Ltd
130 Flaska Drive
Markham, Ontario L6G 1B8
(Orders: Tel: 800 268-4178
         416 470-6739)

Australia
Blackwell Science Pty Ltd
54 University Street
Carlton, Victoria 3053
(Orders: Tel: 03 347-5552)

A catalogue record for this title
is available from the British Library

ISBN 0-632-03811-X

Library of Congress
Cataloging in Publication Data

Kanis, John A. (John Anthony), 1944–
    Osteoporosis/John A. Kanis.
        p.   cm.
    Includes bibliographical references
and index.
    ISBN 0-632-03811-X
    1. Osteoporosis. I. Title.
    [DNLM: 1. Osteoporosis—
prevention & control.
    2. Osteoporosis—therapy.
    3. Osteoporosis—etiology.
    WE 250 K160 1994]
    RC931.O73K36 1994
    616.7'16—dc20

Contents

Foreword

Osteoporosis is thought to be one of the leading causes of disability and loss of independence in our aging Canadian population. Because of this, it has been selected as one of two major health topics for public health research initiatives by the Canadian government. There are actually very few available data on osteoporosis incidence and costs in Canada, but what little we know suggests it is an extremely important problem. The most recent estimate by Statistics Canada was approximately 25 000 hip fractures in 1989–90, with an estimated direct cost of acute medical care approaching $400 million. There is some indication that the age-adjusted incidence of hip fractures is increasing in this country, and it is projected that there will be approximately 30 000 first-time hip fractures per year in Canada by the year 2006. There are no Canadian studies of the financial and social cost of the long-term care of people with hip fractures or the even more common problem of vertebral fractures. Increased awareness of osteoporosis by physicians, government, and the general public is needed to develop effective programs for treatment prevention.

Not too long ago, it was often said that our knowledge of treatment and prevention of osteoporosis had not advanced because the people most commonly affected, women over the age of 60, were in a group which politicians and medical researchers tended to ignore. While there may have been more than a little truth to that statement, there were other problems preventing the improvement of the state of knowledge about osteoporosis: (i) there were no readily available methods of measuring bone mass, either for diagnosis or measuring effectiveness of treatment; (ii) there were almost no centres capable of examining the effect of therapy on the process of bone remodelling at a cellular or biochemical level; (iii) our ability to study bone cells in culture was in its infancy; and (iv) our knowledge of how to properly conduct clinical trials was rudimentary. However, osteoporosis research has benefited greatly from a number of dramatic changes in medicine which have occurred in the past 10–15 years. Measurement of bone mass has become widely available, as have bone pathology techniques and biochemical markers of bone turnover.

Basic studies of bone biology have demonstrated the estrogen receptor in bone cells, and molecular geneticists have even found evidence for an 'osteoporosis gene'. A large number of well-designed clinical trials of a variety of highly potent agents to treat or prevent osteoporosis are in progress, as well as studies of determinants of peak bone mass and modifiable risk factors for osteoporosis.

These are exciting times for all of us interested in bone disease, as it seems that every day we hear of new and important advances being made at all levels of research, from the most basic studies of bone biology to clinical trials and epidemiologic surveys. This book, by one of the most prominent thought leaders in the field of osteoporosis is a very readable and thorough summary of the present state of our knowledge of this disorder. In addition to his own considerable research contributions, Dr Kanis has long been recognized for his ability to review the field and bring out the key points for the practising clinician, and this monograph is no exception.

The Osteoporosis Society of Canada is committed to the promotion of education and research in this area, and is therefore pleased to help promote this book.

DAVID A. HANLEY
Professor and Head
Division of Endocrinology and Metabolism
Department of Medicine
Foothills Hospital and the University of Calgary
Chairperson, Scientific Advisory Board
Osteoporosis Society of Canada

Preface

The clinical significance of osteoporosis arises from the fractures that occur. They are very disabling and in the case of hip fracture are an important cause of death. In many countries, osteoporosis is the most common metabolic bone disease. In others, the increasing life expectancy and changes in lifestyle indicate that the problems of osteoporosis will markedly affect the majority in years to come. The clinical consequences of osteoporosis are fractures, of which hip fracture is the most serious, both for the individual and health-care systems. About 1.6 million hip fractures are estimated to occur each year or one every 20 seconds. Because of continued improvements in health care and life expectancy the number of elderly will increase markedly. Conservative estimates suggest that in 60 years, the number of hip fractures worldwide will rise to more than 6 million, so that osteoporosis has a substantial and ever increasing economic significance.

There is much information on the pathophysiology and the treatment of osteoporosis. Indeed, there are a number of treatments available and many new therapeutic agents are being tested. With some possible exceptions, treatment today prevents the progression of the disease rather than curing it, so that in order to decrease the health-care burden of fragility fractures, intervention is best undertaken as early as possible in the natural history of the disease.

The major problem in the management of the disorder today is that the diagnosis of osteoporosis is most frequently made only when a fracture has occurred. Bone loss is usually very slow and asymptomatic until a fracture has occurred. This means that the disorder has usually been present for many years before it is diagnosed. For this reason, early recognition of osteoporosis is important if significant inroads are to be made in tackling the problem. Responsibility for the care of osteoporotic patients lies with the primary-care physician and in some countries with physicians and surgeons with a particular sub-speciality interest. The aims of this book are to provide an aid to the early diagnosis and management of osteoporosis – a largely preventable disease.

Acknowledgements

I am most grateful to Wendy Pontefract for typing the manuscript and to Monique Benéton for extensive proof reading. My thanks also to Amanda Ryde and Charlie Hamlyn from Blackwell Science for their enthusiasm and support. Constraints on space mean that the contributions of many investigators are not acknowledged and I trust that they view this as a sin of omission rather than commission.

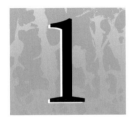

Osteoporosis and its consequences

The currently accepted definition of osteoporosis is: 'A systemic skeletal disease characterized by low bone mass and micro-architectural deterioration of bone tissue, with a consequent increase in bone fragility and susceptibility to fracture risk' (Anon, 1993).

A working definition of osteoporosis is a useful starting point. Unfortunately, like many terms, osteoporosis defies a completely accurate description. It is traditionally thought of as a generalized disorder of bone in which bone mass is reduced, but this framework is unsatisfactory for several reasons. It omits focal causes of osteoporosis such as neoplasia, immobilization or fracture. These are of some importance since there have been marked advances in our understanding of the pathophysiology and treatment of these causes of osteoporosis. Conversely, it includes disorders where we have limited knowledge of pathophysiology and treatment, such as osteogenesis imperfecta.

Osteoporosis (or porous bone) is commonly defined in terms of the amount of bone present, but many other factors may contribute to skeletal fragility, whilst fractures are the acknowledged sequelae of osteoporosis. Moreover, other factors contribute to fracture risk, such as falls. The osteoporotic skeleton can be likened to a fragile vase in the sense that the vase will not break unless it is tipped over. Similarly, the skeleton will not break unless subject to stresses. For these reasons, definitions of osteoporosis variously emphasize bone mass or other determinants of skeletal fragility, the degree of trauma or the response to trauma.

These different approaches arise because of the multifactorial nature of the disease. This chapter summarizes some of the individual components of risk (reviewed in greater detail in subsequent pages) in order to provide a framework for its definition and thereafter describes the fractures which are the consequences of osteoporosis.

Osteoporosis and fracture

The clinical significance of osteoporosis lies in the fractures which arise, and for this reason it is acknowledged as a major problem of health care. Common sites of fracture are the spine, wrist and hip, but when bone loss occurs, all sites are at high risk. Osteoporotic fractures occurring at the spine and the forearm are associated with significant morbidity, but the most serious consequences arise in patients with hip fracture, which is associated with a significant

increase in mortality (15–20%), particularly in elderly men and women. Hip fractures account for more than 20% of the orthopaedic beds in the United Kingdom, in Scandinavia and several other countries (Royal College of Physicians, 1989). In 1985, there were 47 000 hip fractures in England and Wales and this accounted for a higher bed occupancy than many other common disorders including breast cancer and diabetes.

There are many statistics available to describe the impact of osteoporosis on our society. These include the incidence of different types of fracture, the frequency of low bone mineral density (BMD), and the medical and indirect cost of fractures. Such statistics give little indication of the personal risks from osteoporosis, an approach which can be overcome to some extent by the consideration of lifetime risk. For example, what is the risk of a hip fracture if you happen to be born a woman and live to the age of 50 years? The remaining lifetime risk of hip fracture in white women from the United States is 17.5% and similar estimates of risk are found in most Western European countries. The risk for other types of osteoporotic fractures are nearly as high (Table 1.1), so that the combined risk is 40%. Thus

four in 10 women will sustain one or more osteoporotic fractures in their lifetime. This estimate is conservative since it only takes into account vertebral fractures which come to clinical attention, so that the true risk of fracture is higher. In comparison, risks for men are about one-third of those in women, and are even lower for forearm fractures.

These indices of risk compare with a lifetime risk of 9% for breast cancer and 40% for cardiovascular disease for women at the age of 50 years. These data indicate the widespread prevalence of the disorder in our society.

Determinants of fracture

The incidence of osteoporotic fractures increases with age in both sexes, and a great deal of evidence indicates that this is causally related to changes in the amount of bone tissue present in the skeleton. The size of bones does not decrease with age, indeed the width of tubular bones may increase. Rather, the porosity of the bones increases so that the proportion of bone occupied by bone tissue is decreased. This is traditionally described as a decrease in bone mass or a decrease in the BMD and is commonly paraphrased as

a decrease in bone density, though the term is inaccurate.

Table 1.1 Estimated lifetime fracture risk in women (95% confidence intervals) from Rochester at the age of 50 years

Fracture site	Women	Men
Proximal femur	17.5 (16.8−18.2)	6.0 (5.6−6.5)
Vertebral*	15.6 (14.8−16.3)	5.0 (4.6−5.4)
Distal forearm	16.0 (15.7−16.7)	2.5 (2.2−3.1)
Any of the above	39.7 (38.7−40.6)	13.1 (12.4−13.7)

* Clinically diagnosed fractures. (From Melton *et al.*, 1991.)

The factors involved in the amount of bone present, and hence the risk of fractures in adult life, are the peak bone mass attained in early adulthood and the amount of bone lost, for example, during the course of disease or after the menopause. The determinants of peak bone mass and bone loss differ (see Chapter 2) and both may be affected by disease, environmental factors and by treatment. In the average menopausal woman, the contribution of peak bone mass and postmenopausal bone loss to the risk of fracture are approximately equal at the age of 75 years, when, for example, most hip fractures occur.

Loss of skeletal strength

The loss of bone that occurs in osteoporosis is associated with several other structural and qualitative abnormalities which contribute to the loss of skeletal strength. These include changes in the turnover of bone to repair fatigue damage and the loss of connectivity of the trabecular elements which comprise cancellous bone. These and other abnormalities are collectively termed alterations in the quality of bone (Fig. 1.1), and although they contribute to skeletal weakness,

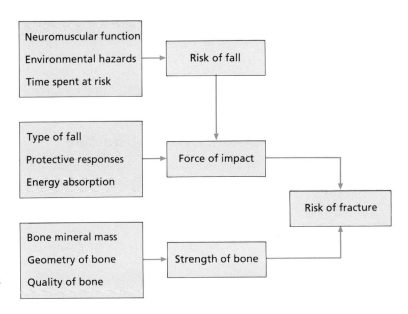

Fig. 1.1 Schema to show the determinants of fracture risk.

some of these changes in the quality of bone are the direct consequence of bone loss itself. Over and above this, bone mass is not the sole determinant of fracture risk. For any given bone mass, the risk of fracture is greater in the elderly in part because of an increased tendency to fall and a decreased ability to react appropriately to diminish the force of impacts. This is true in the case of Colles' fracture at the forearm and for the vast majority of hip fractures, but not quite so true for vertebral crush fractures which may occur as a result of everyday activities such as bending, coughing or lifting. Thus the contribution of skeletal and extraskeletal factors varies in different fracture types and indeed for a given fracture between individuals.

Differences in bone mass

Despite this multiplicity of factors, attention is focused on bone mass rather than other determinants of fracture risk, largely because of the variety of non-invasive techniques that are available for the measurement of bone mineral content (BMC) or BMD (see Chapter 5). Indeed, differences in bone mass account in some measure for the differing risk of fracture between men and women. Women have a lower peak bone mass than men at many skeletal sites. In addition to a lower peak bone mass, women have a greater age-related loss, which is accelerated at the menopause. The rate of bone loss is approximately 1% per annum in men beginning from middle age whereas in women higher rates of bone loss (2−4% per annum) occur in the first 5−10 years following the menopause due to gonadal deficiency. Women also have a longer life expectancy than men so they are exposed to a lower bone mass and falls for longer periods.

Men vs. women

Although differences in bone mass are of importance, there are other factors which account for the differences between the sexes. For example, elderly women fall more often than men and differences in bone mass may not explain completely the different patterns of risk that are found between cultures and races. Notwithstanding, of the various factors which contribute to fracture risk, the amount of bone present is the sole factor which can be measured accurately before fractures occur. For this reason, osteoporosis is often defined in terms of the amount of bone present in an individual.

What is osteoporosis?

The meaning of the term osteoporosis has been the subject of some debate (Kanis, 1990). To the epidemiologist, the term is often used to describe a clinical outcome such as a hip fracture. However, hip fractures occur in healthy individuals due to excessive trauma, so that an appreciation of skeletal fragility is appropriate to any definition. From the point of view of the disease process, osteoporosis can be defined as a disorder in which there is a diminution of bone mass without a detectable change in the ratio of mineralized to non-mineralized bone (to exclude osteomalacia). In recent years broader definitions have been utilized which capture the concept of a hetero-geneity of skeletal and extraskeletal factors in the causation of fractures.

Osteoporosis and
fracture

Future definitions may take more account of extraskeletal risk factors but are likely to maintain the distinction between the disease (reduced bone mass) and the clinical complication (fracture). An appropriate analogy is the distinction between hypertension and stroke. Hypertension is certainly an important cause of stroke, but many strokes occur in the absence of hypertension. In the same way, fractures occur in the absence of osteoporosis although in the presence of osteoporosis the risk of fracture is very high.

DIAGNOSING OSTEOPOROSIS

Fracture threshold

The high accuracy of techniques to measure bone mineral mass makes them appropriate for use as a diagnostic test for osteoporosis. Several approaches have been utilized to diagnose osteoporosis on the basis of bone mineral measurements (Kanis, 1990). The most straightforward is to define a fracture threshold, namely the cut-off for BMD which captures most patients with osteoporotic fractures. This can be variously and arbitrarily set, for example at the mean or 1 or 2 standard deviations (SD) above the mean value of patients with osteoporotic fracture, or at a set point below the mean of the young adult reference range. The setting of the fracture threshold depends not only on the site measured and technique used but also on other factors such as the site of interest, age and sex.

In adult women, the cut-off value of 2.5 SD below the average of the healthy young adult range is appropriate to satisfy many of these criteria, particularly for hip fracture (Newton-John & Morgan, 1970). More than one cut-off can be chosen to denote the severity of disease. This permits four general diagnostic categories to be established for adult women, and the following have been accepted by the European Foundation for Osteoporosis and Bone Disease, the National Osteoporosis Foundation of the United States and the World Health Organization (WHO, 1994).

Working definition

1 Normal. A value for BMD or BMC not more than 1 SD below the average value of young adults.
2 A low bone mass (or osteopenia). A value for BMD or BMC more than 1 SD below the young adult average, but not more than 2.5 SD below.
3 Osteoporosis. A value for BMD or BMC more than 2.5 SD below the young adult average value.
4 Severe osteoporosis. (established osteoporosis). A value for BMD or BMC more than 2.5 SD below the young adult average value and the presence of one or more fragility fractures.

The diagnostic categories above identify approximately 30% of postmenopausal women as having osteoporosis using measurements made at the spine, hip or forearm. This is approximately equivalent to the lifetime risk of fracture at any of these sites. When measurements are made at the one site alone, then the prevalence is 15–20%, comparable to the lifetime risk of a single osteoporotic fracture such as a hip fracture.

Because the distribution of values for BMD in the young healthy population is Gaussian, the incidence of osteoporosis increases exponentially after the age of 50 years (Fig. 1.2) as is also the case for many osteoporosis-related fractures. Since values for BMC or BMD and for fracture risk are both continuously distributed in the population, there is no absolute criterion in the absence of fracture that can delineate an individual with the disease from one without. In this sense, the concept of disease differs from, say, breast cancer

Osteoporosis increases exponentially with age

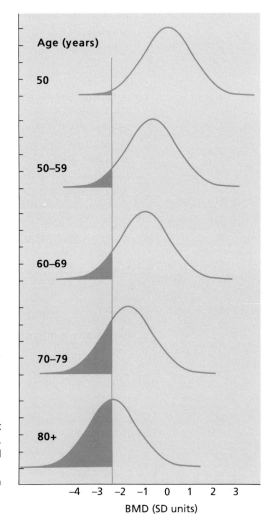

Fig. 1.2 Bone mineral density (BMD) in women at different ages and the prevalence of osteoporosis. The graph shows that BMD is normally distributed at all ages but decreases progressively with age. The proportion of patients with osteoporosis with a BMD 2.5 SD units or less than the young adult reference mean increases exponentially with age.

where the individual either has or does not have the disease, even though it may be variously clinically overt or covert. For this reason, there is an overlap between BMD in populations with or without fracture, irrespective of the technique used and the cut-off chosen and the site of measurements. Again, the analogy to hypertension is appropriate.

Diagnostic use of BMD

The use of BMD as a diagnostic test can be utilized to determine whether a fracture is due to osteoporosis or whether a patient at high risk (for example, on long-term corticosteroid treatment) has osteoporosis. The indications for the use of mineral measurements in this way are reviewed in Chapter 5.

Different criteria than those pertaining to adult women should be applied in the case of men and younger individuals before skeletal maturity. In men, the risk of fracture is substantially lower for bone mineral measurements within their own reference range so that a criteria of 3 SD may be more appropriate for the diagnosis of osteoporosis.

PREDICTING OSTEOPOROTIC FRACTURES

A further use of bone mineral measurement is in the assessment of risk, namely to assess the probability of future fractures. The accuracy of the test in this context is the ability of bone mineral measurement at any one site to predict the probability of a future osteoporotic fracture at that site or elsewhere. This application is of critical importance in developing treatment and preventive strategies. This use contrasts with the use of bone mineral measurement to diagnose osteoporosis, where accuracy is the ability to measure BMD at the site measured, or at other sites of biological relevance. The test is thus utilized to elicit a risk factor in the context of risk prediction. There are once again useful analogies with other diseases such as hypertension where blood pressure is used clinically as a predictor of risk (Table 1.2).

Prognostic use of BMD

The test only has practical value if there is an adequate gradient of risk associated with a reduction in BMD. The greater increase in risk for a finite reduction in BMD, the more useful the test, since more

Table 1.2 Examples of the distinction between risk factors and disease

Disease	Risk factor	Clinical expression
Coronary artery disease	Hypercholesterolaemia	Myocardial infarction
Hypertension	High blood pressure	Stroke
Osteoporosis	Low bone mineral density	Fracture
Gout	Hyperuricaemia	Arthritis

individuals will be identified correctly to be at either high or low risk.

Gradient of fracture risk

The performance of the various techniques are summarized in Chapter 5, but suffice to say that the gradient of risk of fracture with bone mineral measurement is somewhat steeper than those reported for serum cholesterol or hypertension and the risk of coronary artery disease in men. For example, in a large study of risk factor interventions, there was approximately a 1.5-fold increase in the risk of death from coronary artery disease with each SD decrease in serum cholesterol or increase in diastolic blood pressure after adjusting for confounding factors (Fig. 1.3). This gradient of risk is also similar to that reported for systolic blood pressure and risk of stroke-associated mortality (Khaw *et al.*, 1984). In contrast, there is a two- to fourfold increase in fracture risk with each SD decrease in bone mineral, depending on the site of measurement and the techniques used.

Increase in fracture risk

The consequences of osteoporosis

Bone loss causes no symptoms

There is no evidence that bone loss itself causes any symptoms and progressive bone loss has therefore been called 'the silent epidemic' or 'silent thief'. The morbidity arises largely from the fractures which are sustained, but not all fractures are due to osteoporosis. In many Western countries the frequency of all fractures is similar among men and women and a minority are associated with osteoporosis. There are, however, large differences in the age at which fractures occur. In men three-quarters of all fractures occur under the age of 45 years, whereas in women three-quarters occur after this age. In women over the age of 45 years the vast majority of fractures are attributable to osteoporosis (Kanis & Pitt, 1992; Melton, 1993).

Age and fracture risk

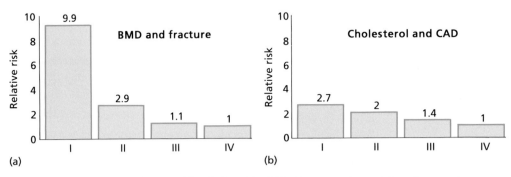

Fig. 1.3 (a) Relative risk of hip fracture estimated from forearm bone mineral density (BMD) in a cohort of 399 women aged 40–70 years followed up for 10 years. (From Gardsell *et al.*, 1993.) The relative risk in the population is shown by quartiles of BMD. The 25% of the population with the highest BMD is accorded a risk of 1.0. (b) Shows the change in relative risk for coronary artery disease (CAD) according to quartiles of serum cholesterol in men. (From Neaton *et al.*, 1992.)

In men the incidence rate of fractures increases substantially after the age of 75 years whereas in women an increase is seen after the age of 45 years. In women, increases up to the age of 65 years are due largely to an increase in forearm fractures. After this age, hip fractures assume a greater importance both in men and women, and from 85 years of age onwards the hip is the most common site of fracture. Between the ages of 5 and 14 years, approximately one-third of fractures require hospital admission (Kanis & Pitt, 1992), but among the elderly the majority of all patients with fractures are hospitalized.

There are a number of other types of fractures which increase exponentially with age, though they are quantitatively less important than hip fracture, both in socioeconomic terms and in the morbidity they cause. Sites include the humerus, ankle, pelvis, ribs and spine. With the exception of pelvic fractures the increase in risk with age is less than for hip fracture (Fig. 1.4).

OSTEOPOROTIC FRACTURES

The number of fractures due to osteoporosis is difficult to quantify accurately. One method is to assess the excess fracture rate compared to the young adult community. In men, for example, the incidence of all fractures increases from the age of 65 years. The excess number of fractures from this age in England and Wales amounts to 17 000 fractures per year excluding vertebral fractures (Kanis & Pitt, 1992). In women, fractures increase progressively from the age of 45 years, and the excess number of fractures after this age is 97 000 per year. Thus, at least 114 000 fractures per annum are associated with aging, of which the vast majority (85%) occur in women. These figures are an underestimate since they take no account of vertebral fractures. If

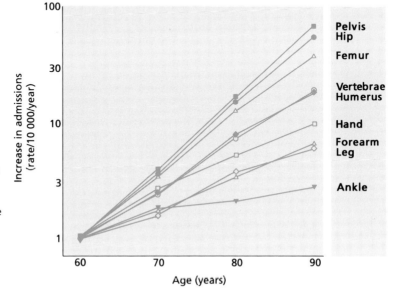

Fig. 1.4 Rate of increase in admission for different fractures by age in women from the Trent Region of England. Rates are standardized at a value of 1 at the age of 60. Note the logarithmic rise in rates for all the sites shown. (From Kanis & Pitt, 1992)

vertebral fractures are included then these numbers might double, though an uncertain proportion of them would be asymptomatic. This estimate is similar to those from the United States if differences in population demography are taken into account (Phillips *et al.*, 1988).

It is assumed that fractures, which increase with age, are attributable to osteoporosis. This is not invariably true. The relative contribution of osteoporosis and age from a prospective study in women aged 65 years or more show that fractures of the ankle, elbow, finger and face occur independently of bone mass, representing 26% of all fractures. Thus, osteoporotic fractures in this sense account for the vast majority of fractures.

The most common osteoporotic fractures in women comprise Colles' fracture of the wrist, vertebral compression fractures and fractures of the neck of femur. The lifetime risk of these fractures in women is at least 30% and probably closer to 40% (see Table 1.1), although it varies from country to country.

HIP FRACTURE

The most severe osteoporotic fracture is hip fracture, which typically results from falling from the standing position, but may occur spontaneously. It is usually painful, and nearly always necessitates hospitalization. For this reason, estimates of incidence, costs and other consequences are better documented than for other osteoporotic fractures.

The increase in risk for hip fracture with age can be described by an exponential curve in most communities, both in men and women. In general, rates are higher in women than in men but this is variable. The lifetime risk varies between countries and in Europe alone the incidence in women varies more than 10-fold (see Chapter 2). Similar variations in risk are found within the United States. There are similar, if less marked, variations in male risk. The average age at presentation with hip fracture is 75 years in England (Royal College of Physicians, 1989), but varies in other countries depending on the demography of the region studied and the type of hip fracture.

Most hip fractures in the elderly arise from moderate trauma defined as a fall from a standing height to level ground. There is a continuous debate whether patients fall and break their hip or whether they break their hip and fall. Most hip fractures arise by direct impact over the hip and the risk of fracture is substantially lower if the fall is not directly onto the hip (Cummings & Nevitt, 1989). This suggests that the fall is important. On the other hand, some patients do describe pain on bearing weight for several days or weeks before falling, perhaps due to an incomplete fracture at that site. Thus, a combination of factors may operate in a minority of patients.

The pain due to hip fracture varies considerably, probably related to differences in the degree of trauma, blood loss, etc. In most patients, the diagnosis is obvious because of pain, inability to rise and external rotation of the leg. The diagnosis is confirmed by X-ray. Some undisplaced fractures may, however, not be visible on radiographs. In such patients, further X-rays or bone scintigraphy may be helpful. The detection of undisplaced hip fractures facilitates surgical management and improves the prognosis.

Types of hip fracture

History

There are broadly speaking two types of hip fracture, cervical fractures and lateral or trochanteric fractures, and they have a somewhat different natural history and treatment. Trochanteric fractures are more characteristically osteoporotic and the secular trend in the incidence of hip fracture is greater for trochanteric than for cervical fractures. In many countries they occur with equal frequency, though the average age of patients with trochanteric fractures is approximately 5 years older than for cervical fractures.

Treatment

Undisplaced cervical fractures are usually treated by internal fixation with multiple pins. There are various options for displaced fractures: open reduction and internal fixation is commonly undertaken in the young, but avascular necrosis and non-union may require a second operation and hip replacement. For this reason, elderly patients are often treated with a prosthetic replacement which also permits immediate mobilization. Intertrochanteric fractures are generally treated by internal fixation unless there are very strong contraindications to surgery. Healing does occur with traction, but this requires prolonged bed rest with its attendant hazards. The most commonly used fixation devices utilize a sliding screw and plate.

Traction

Fractures appear to heal normally in osteoporotic patients but there is a high degree of morbidity and appreciable mortality dependent in part on age, treatment and associated morbidity. Complications may arise because of immobility before or after diagnosis. Some elderly patients living alone are unable to seek assistance and may lie for hours or days before being discovered. This increases the risks of hypothermia, pneumonia and pressure sores.

Immobility

The duration of acute hospitalization varies according to orthopaedic practice and the availability of facilities for postoperative rehabilitation. Average hospital admission times are 20–30 days.

Surgical complications

Complications arise from the fracture, surgery and comorbidity. Surgical complications occur in 30% of patients and include nonunion or delayed union, avascular necrosis of the femoral head and loosening of prosthetic implants (Lips & Obrant, 1991). Despite effective surgical management long-term morbidity is also high. When functional status before fractures is taken into account, 30% of women become functionally dependent after fracture, of whom the majority (two-thirds) require nursing home care (Table 1.3). Approximately 25% regain their former mobility whereas over half require assistance in walking or other activities and the remainder are unable to maintain usual everyday activities. Thus a minority of patients regain their former mobility. As expected, morbidity increases with age. A minority of patients will sustain a second hip fracture. The

Nursing home care

Table 1.3 Hip fracture outcome according to functional status before fracture. (Modified from Chrischilles *et al.*, 1991)

	Probability of outcome after fracture		
Status before fracture	Independent	Dependent	Nursing home
Independent	0.74	0.18	0.08
Dependent	—	0.50	0.50
Nursing home	—	—	1.00

lifetime risk for a further hip fracture is about 8% after a trochanteric fracture. It is higher for cervical fracture (12%) largely because these patients are younger, on average by 5 years or so, than patients with trochanteric fractures.

Mortality

Mortality following hip fracture is appreciable. Figures differ according to differences in populations studied, but range at 1 year from 12 to 40%. The large range reflects the heterogeneity of case sampling and the difficulty in establishing the cause of death in patients who are elderly and have other disorders. Mortality is higher among patients managed conservatively, but there is likely to be considerable selection bias in favour of surgical intervention for the healthier individuals.

The mortality from hip fracture expressed as that in excess of a population of the same age and sex but without fractures amounts to 10–30%. It is caused both by the complications that arise following immobilization and surgery, and by the comorbidity associated with hip fracture, because hip fracture often affects the less healthy segments of society. The excess mortality is greatest within the first 6 months of fracture. In one series of 246 patients with an average age of 75 years, the observed mortality following hip fracture, adjusted for age and sex, was 2.7 times that expected in the first year. After the second year, this dropped to 1.5 indicating that the effects of hip fracture on mortality occur mainly in the first year after fracture (White *et al.*, 1987), but that thereafter comorbidity is still an important factor. As expected, the deaths attributable to hip fracture increase with age.

Years of life lost

Because hip fractures occur predominantly in the elderly, the years of life lost are less than that for many other common diseases. A recent estimate suggested that hip fracture accounted for 9.2 years of life/1000 women compared to 20 years for breast cancer, 29 years for stroke and 73 years for heart disease (Eiskjaer *et al.*, 1992).

VERTEBRAL FRACTURE

Vertebral fractures form an integral component of the osteoporotic syndrome. They are classified as central, wedge, or a crush fracture involving the whole vertebra. Wedging is more common at the an-

Classification

terior than the posterior aspect of the vertebra (see Chapter 5). Fractures often occur spontaneously or as a result of minimal trauma such as during coughing or lifting. As might be expected, high-energy trauma is more common as a cause of vertebral fracture in men than in women (40 vs. 7%), and low-energy trauma assumes progressively greater importance with advancing age (Cooper *et al.*, 1992a). Vertebral fractures show a consistent predilection for the mid-dorsal kyphosis (T7–8) and the thoracolumbar region (Cooper *et al.*, 1992a). The frequency of multiple fractures is approximately half that of single fractures.

Predilection

There are a number of problems which cannot presently be resolved when considering the impact of the vertebral fracture syndrome (Kanis & McCloskey, 1992). Most non-vertebral fractures are clinically obvious and consistently give rise to morbidity, but in the case of vertebral fracture, problems arise in defining the presence or absence of fracture. There is no general agreement about the criteria for the radiographic definition of vertebral fracture, so that reliable data are not ·available on their incidence in the general population. The incidence is also difficult to determine because many vertebral fractures may be asymptomatic, or at least without sufficient symptoms to initiate investigations concerning the cause of back pain. Thus, the proportion of vertebral fractures causing disability is unknown, but is commonly thought to be low. A further problem is that the major manifestation of osteoporosis is back pain, but this is non-specific. Indeed, back pain is so common that, at least up to the age of 70 years, it is more likely when present to be due to other reasons.

Defining vertebral fracture

Prevalence and incidence

It is not possible to give firm estimates of the prevalence or incidence of vertebral fractures largely because of the differing criteria used for their definition (see Chapters 5 and 7). The less stringent cut-offs yield high estimates of prevalence or incidence, but may not be of clinical relevance. More stringent cut-offs give lower estimates but may miss deformities of significance. The lowest rates are expected if crush fracture only were scored (rather than wedging). For example, a survey of 70-year-old women in Denmark identified 21% with existing vertebral fractures (Jensen *et al.*, 1982), but only about a quarter had crush fractures.

One-fifth of women over 75 years

For these reasons the apparent prevalence of established vertebral osteoporosis depends on the criteria used and differs markedly between series. The frequency among women in England and Wales utilizing two quantitative criteria ranges between 256 000 and 565 000 and perhaps provide upper and lower estimates, but still gives a two-fold range of prevalence (Kanis & McCloskey, 1992). Estimates from the United States suggest a prevalence of 25% among women aged 50 years and over (Cooper *et al.*, 1992a).

There are few prospective studies of the incidence of vertebral fracture. On the assumption that vertebral deformities do not heal in adults, the prevalence of vertebral fracture gives the cumulative incidence when mortality is taken into account. The estimated incidence calculated in this way rises exponentially with age (Melton *et al.*, 1989). Although the absolute incidence varies according to the criteria employed, the slope with age is less variable. The risk of vertebral fracture increases 15–30-fold in women between the ages of 50 and 90 years. This compares with a 50-fold increase in the case of hip fracture (see Fig. 1.4; Kanis & Pitt, 1992).

Even less is known of the prevalence or incidence of vertebral osteoporosis in men. Several surveys in Europe suggest that the prevalence among men up to the age of 60 years is higher than among women, presumably related to a more traumatic lifestyle. Thereafter the prevalence increases with age but the slope with age is approximately half that of women. There are few studies of the incidence of vertebral fractures among men. They suggest that the incidence of vertebral fracture over the age of 60 years is approximately half that in women (Cooper *et al.*, 1992a).

Symptomatic vertebral fractures

The consequences of vertebral fracture include kyphosis, back pain and loss of height. The morbidity in the general community is not well characterized, but is likely to be under-reported. New crush fractures may give rise to severe back pain. They often occur during everyday activities such as bending, lifting, coughing or rising from a chair. Falls are less common as a cause. Where pain occurs, this may be sudden and often causes patients to go to bed or immediately consult a doctor. In others the onset of pain is gradual over several days. It is not known whether this represents progressive incremental damage to the vertebral body, but this seems a plausible explanation. Back pain commonly radiates anteriorly to give rise to girdle pain corresponding to the vertebral level affected, and it may be unilateral.

Pain is usually well localized at the specific vertebral level. It is associated with limitation of back movements and is characteristically increased with sitting or standing, and relieved by bed rest. Pain may be exquisite and exacerbated by simple activities such as coughing, sneezing and defaecation. Characteristic sites are the mid-thoracic and upper lumbar sites, in contrast to the common sites for disc prolapse. Ileus, loss of appetite and abdominal distention may occur, perhaps due to retroperitoneal haemorrhage at lower thoracic and lumbar sites.

Tenderness over bony sites is not a feature. Bone pain at the affected level may be elicited by percussion over the fracture site but considerable paravertebral muscle spasm may occur which gives rise to tenderness on palpation. Pain characteristically decreases in severity over several weeks or months, and it may resolve thereafter. During this period there may be limitation of back movements, particularly

Exponential increase in incidence

Incidence in men

Consequences

Pain

Pain usually decreases with time

in flexion. An uncertain proportion of patients may be left with chronic residual pain and disability. On the other hand, some patients give no history of episodes of acute back pain but present with chronic pain, whereas others may have no complaints other than loss of height.

The presence of a symptomatic crush fracture heralds further fractures, and has been shown to be an independent risk factor (Table 1.4). Over 10 years, more than 85% of patients will have recurrent fractures, and three-quarters will lose more than 10 cm in height (Urist, 1973). Further fractures may or may not be associated with further acute pain. Chronic pain is usually relieved by bed rest. Loss of height, a dorsal kyphosis and back pain are the major features of recurrent .vertebral fractures. Loss of height can be approximated

Assessing height loss

from the discrepancy between the standing height and the arm span. Chronic neurological features, such as persistent nerve root pain, are less frequent and paraparesis or spinal cord syndromes are rare.

When a thoracic kyphosis is marked, it requires the patient to hyperextend the neck and may give rise to neck pain and muscle fatigue so that the chin habitually rests on the sternum. Kyphosis

Kyphosis

also reduces the thoracic volume, impairing total lung volume and exercise tolerance. As the thoracic cage descends it may impact onto the pelvic brim, and commonly causes pain as well as distress because of the cosmetic effect on body shape. The reduced abdominal volume causes the abdominal contents to protrude, and characteristically gives rise to creases on the anterior abdominal wall and hiatus hernia (Fig. 1.5).

Among patients with symptoms, pain is most commonly experienced while standing and during physical stress, particularly bending (Leidig et al., 1990). The symptoms are, however, variable and not sufficiently specific to aid in diagnosis. Whereas pain may be the most prominent symptom, it seems likely that other morbidity is under-recognized. Patients do have limitation of movement which impacts onto daily living. A problem often reported by patients is

Fear of falling

fear of falling, which may be as disabling as the fracture itself in terms of its impact on daily activities and the feeling of well-being. Chronic pain may contribute to depressed mood, and kyphosis impairs the ability to perform simple tasks (e.g., lying flat in bed or putting

Table 1.4 Relative risk of fracture at the sites shown in women (95% confidence intervals) with symptomatic vertebral fracture. (From Cooper et al., 1991)

Site	Relative risk
Hip	2.2 (1.7−2.8)
Distal forearm	2.2 (1.7−2.8)
Proximal humerus	3.5 (3.5−4.6)

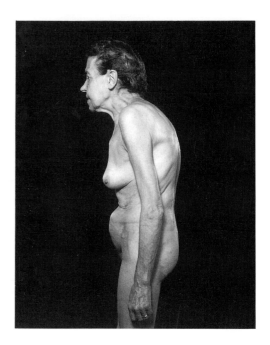

Fig. 1.5 Clinical photograph of a patient with multiple compression fractures due to osteoporosis. Note the loss of waistline, the protruberant abdomen and the anterior crease on the abdomen.

on shoes). Kyphosis also causes considerable distress due to the effect on appearance and ability to dress smartly. All these factors tend to make patients reluctant to go outdoors and interact socially. The few studies which have attempted to quantify morbidity suggest that this lies midway between that found in health and that following hip fracture (Fig. 1.6). Scores for morbidity are significantly higher in patients with more than a single crush fracture (Leidig *et al.*, 1990).

Sickness impact scores

When sickness impact scores are assessed by age, osteoporotic women between the ages of 55 and 64 years have scores expected of healthy women aged 75 years or more.

Because the incidence of vertebral fracture cannot be accurately quantified, the proportion of patients with vertebral osteoporosis who suffer morbid consequences is also unknown, but several esti-

Fig. 1.6 Morbidity in patients with osteoporotic fractures assessed using the sickness impact profile (SIP). Patients with vertebral fractures had a score midway between that associated with hip fracture and that in age- and sex-matched controls. (From Kanis & McCloskey, 1992.)

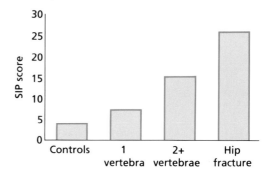

mates suggest that the incidence of symptomatic fractures is about half that estimated from the prevalence of fractures (Kanis & McCloskey, 1992) but is lower when more sensitive quantitative indices of vertebral deformity are utilized.

Increased mortality

Although atraumatic vertebral fracture is very rarely fatal, mortality is increased in patients with vertebral fracture (Cooper et al., 1993). Low bone density is also associated with an increased mortality (Browner et al., 1991). Indeed, osteoporosis may be as strong a predictor of mortality as blood pressure or serum cholesterol. The reasons do not relate to the fracture itself, since, unlike hip fracture, there is no excess mortality immediately after fracture: rather the increased risk is continuous. The reasons for excess mortality are a higher number of deaths from chronic obstructive airways disease, gastrointestinal disease and infection. Deaths from stroke or coronary artery disease are less than expected.

FRACTURES OF THE DISTAL FOREARM

Cause

Over 80% of forearm fractures are at the distal radius, usually Colles' fracture. They are usually caused by a fall on the outstretched hand. Although they occur in women before as well as after the menopause, bone mass is reduced in premenopausal women with Colles' fracture, indicating the importance of peak bone density in determining susceptibility to this fracture.

Lifetime risk

The incidence in women increases rapidly from the first 5 years of the menopause reaching a peak between the ages of 60 and 70 years. In some series, the incidence flattens off after this age, whereas in others it continues to rise. The lifetime risk of having a Colles' fracture is approximately 15% in European and American women, and about 20% of 70-year-old women have had at least one wrist fracture.

Fractures may variously involve the ulna or radio-ulnar joint depending on the degree of trauma, which is most commonly graded according to the scale of Frykmann. In young women, the disorder is associated with higher degrees of trauma and the degree of bony injury sustained is proportionately more severe.

Consequences

Although fractures of the wrist cause less morbidity than those of the hip, are very rarely fatal and seldom require hospitalization, the consequences are often underestimated. Wrist fractures are painful, usually require one or more reductions and need 4−6 weeks in plaster to establish union. The need for hospitalization rises with age and 70% of patients with Colles' fracture aged 85 years or more require hospitalization. A proportion do not recover immediate function. Prospective studies show that there is a high incidence of algodystrophy after Colles' fracture (30%) which gives rise to pain and tenderness, stiffness, swelling and vasomotor disturbances of the hand and more rarely the frozen shoulder syndrome (see Chapter 4). The disorder commonly resolves spontaneously, but pain and stiffness are a persistent feature. At 1 year after Colles' fracture the majority of patients with algodystrophy will have residual stiffness (Table 1.5). Other complications include malunion giving rise to deformity, shortening of the radius and radio-ulnar joint dislocation. In some patients carpal tunnel syndrome and other neurological compression injuries may occur. If the articular surface of the radiocarpal joint is damaged osteoarthrosis may develop in later life.

Mortality
Several studies suggest that mortality is not higher among women with Colles' fracture than among the general population, and contrasts with the pattern of mortality seen with other osteoporotic fractures.

COSTS OF OSTEOPOROSIS

Factors affecting costs
The total costs of osteoporosis are difficult to assess because they include acute hospital care, loss of working days, chronic care in the home or nursing homes, medication, etc. Estimates of the costs of osteoporosis rest on many assumptions which are difficult to test. Moreover, there is little information which is of value to translate costs from one country to another. The costs of osteoporotic fractures in the United States are estimated at $20 billion annually for a population of 250 million and are escalating rapidly (Melton, 1993). In England and Wales the total cost of osteoporosis is estimated to be £614 million annually for a population of 50 million (Kanis & Pitt, 1992).

The vast majority of these costs are attributable to hip fracture because of the in-patient and nursing home demands on such patients. Hip fractures account for over half of all the osteoporosis-related hospital admissions in the United States in women over the age of 45 years, and even more in England and Wales (Kanis & Pitt, 1992).

Hospital admissions

SECULAR TRENDS

Increase in frequency
In many countries, the frequency of osteoporotic fractures in the community has increased progressively. Part of the explanation is the increased longevity of the population (see Chapter 4). The size of the population at high risk is likely to increase in the future in nearly all countries. In the 25 years from 1985 the overall population in England and Wales will increase by 3%, but the increment in the

Table 1.5 Residual morbidity (%) in patients with algodystrophy complicating Colles' fracture. (Data from Bickerstaff & Kanis, 1994)

Feature	At 3 months	At 6 months	At 1 year
Tenderness	77	55	18
Pain	61	30	14
Vascular instability	91	65	29
Swelling	87	29	12
Stiffness	89	76	65

population over the age of 80 years will be 47% in the case of women and 93% in the case of men (Royal College of Physicians, 1989). Since the risk of fractures increases with age, more and more of the population will be exposed to a high risk. Demographic changes in the United States could cause the number of fractures to double over the next 50 years. The effect is likely to be even greater in Asia.

These demographic changes are not, however, the sole reason for the increased frequency of osteoporotic fracture. The age- and sex-specific incidence of several types of fracture is also increasing. For example, the incidence of hip fracture in Oxford, England, doubled over a 27-year period from the 1950s (Boyce & Vessey, 1985), and similar increases have been seen in other regions of the world (Table 1.6).

Because of differences in the incidence of osteoporotic fractures around the world, differences in secular trends and uncertainties about the incidence of many types of osteoporotic fracture, it is difficult to quantitate the burden of osteoporosis in the world today. This has been attempted for hip fracture, and it has been estimated that about 1.7 million hip fractures occurred worldwide in 1990 (Cooper et al., 1992b). The world population is expected to increase and, because of increasing life-expectancy, the number of elderly individuals will increase even more. On a worldwide basis it is estimated that the number of hip fractures could rise to 6.25 million

by 2050 (Cooper et al., 1992b). These projections assume that age-specific rates will not increase with time. They thus provide very conservative estimates for the future. For example, there were 47 000 hip fractures in England and Wales in 1985, which is expected to increase to 60 000 by the year 2016, solely because of the aging of the community. If, however, age- and sex-specific incidence rates rise as they did between the 1950s and 1980s then this estimate would have to be revised to 117 000 hip fractures. These considerations indicate that the burden of osteoporotic fractures will increase substantially in all communities where life-expectancy or the average length of life of individuals continues to increase.

Table 1.6 Age- and sex-specific incidence for hip fracture (rate/100 000) in Hong Kong in 1966 and 1989. Note the increase in rates at all ages and in both sexes. (From Lau et al., 1990)

Age (years)	Men		Women	
	1966	1989	1966	1989
40–49	6	8	7	3
50–59	16	21	23	25
60–69	71	77	57	113
70–79	224	307	173	507
80+	321	898	716	1327

Reasons for the increase in age- and sex-specific incidence are not known but affect both men and women (see Table 1.6). Possibilities include decreased physical exercise, secular increases in height and changes in environmental factors such as the hardness of surfaces on which falls occur.

References

Anon (1993) Consensus development conference: diagnosis, prophylaxis and treatment of osteoporosis. *Am J Med*; **94**: 646–650.

Bickerstaff DR, Kanis JA (1994) Algodystrophy: an under-recognized complication of minor trauma. *Br J Rheumatol*; **33**: in press.

Boyce WJ, Vessey MP (1985) Rising incidence of fracture of the proximal femur. *Lancet*; **i**: 150–151.

Browner WS, Seelet DG, Vogt TM, Cummings SR (1991) Non-trauma mortality in elderly women with low bone mineral density. *Lancet*; **338**: 355–358.

Chrischilles EA, Butler CD, Davis CS, Wallace RBA (1991) Model of lifetime osteoporosis impact. *Arch Intern Med*; **151**: 2026–2032.

Cooper C, Shah S, Hand DJ *et al.* (1991) Screening for vertebral osteoporosis using individual risk factors. *Osteoporosis Int*; **2**: 48–53.

Cooper C, Atkinson EJ, O'Fallon WM, Melton LJ (1992a) Incidence of clinically diagnosed vertebral fractures: a population-based study in Rochester, Minnesota, 1985–1989. *J Bone Miner Res*; **7**: 221–227.

Cooper C, Campion G, Melton LJ (1992b) Hip fractures in the elderly: a worldwide projection. *Osteoporosis Int*; **2**: 285–289.

Cooper C, Atkinson EJ, Jacobsen SJ, O'Fallon WM (1993) Survival following vertebral fractures. A population-based study. *Am J Epidemiol*; **86**: 247–253.

Cummings SR, Nevitt MC (1989) Epidemiology of hip fractures and falls. In Kleerekoper M, Krane SM (eds). *Clinical Disorders of Bone and Mineral Metabolism*, pp. 231–236. Mary Ann Liebert Inc, Publishers, New York.

Eiskjaer S, Ostgard SE, Jakobsen BW, Jensen J, Lucht U (1992) Years of potential life lost after hip fracture among postmenopausal women. *Acta Orthop Scand*; **63**: 293–296.

Gardsell P, Johnell O, Nilsson BE, Gullberg B (1993) Predicting various fragility fractures in women by forearm bone density. *Calcif Tissue Int*; **52**: 348–353.

Jensen GF, Christiansen C, Boeseen J, Hegedus V, Transbol I (1982) Epidemiology of postmenopausal spinal and long bone fractures: a unifying approach to postmenopausal osteoporosis. *Clin Orthop*; **166**: 75–81.

Kanis JA (1990) Osteoporosis and osteopenia. *J Bone Miner Res*; **5**, 209–211.

Kanis JA, McCloskey EV (1992) The epidemiology of vertebral osteoporosis. *Bone*; **13** (suppl. 2): S1–S10.

Kanis JA, Pitt F (1992) Epidemiology of osteoporosis. *Bone*; **13** (suppl. 1): S7–S15.

Khaw K, Barrett-Connor E, Suarez L, Crique MH (1984) Predictors of stroke associated mortality in the elderly. *Stroke*; **15**: 244–248.

Lau EMC, Cooper C, Wickham C, Donnan S, Barker DJP (1990) Hip fracture in Hong Kong and Britain. *Int J Epidemiol*; **19**: 1119–1121.

Leidig G, Minne HW, Sauer P *et al.* (1990) A study of complaints and their relation to vertebral destruction in patients with osteoporosis. *Bone Miner*; **8**: 217–229.

Lips P, Obrant KJ (1991) The pathogenesis and treatment of hip fractures. *Osteoporosis Int*; **1**: 218–231.

Melton LJ (1993) Hip fractures: a worldwide problem today and tomorrow. *Bone*; **14** (suppl.): 1–8.

Melton LJ, Kan SH, Frye MA, Wahner HW, O'Fallon WM, Riggs BL (1989) Epidemiology of vertebral fractures in women. *Am J Epidemiol*; **129**: 1000–1011.

Melton LJ, Atkinson EJ, O'Fallon WM, Wahner HW, Riggs BL (1991) Long-term fracture risk prediction with bone mineral measurements made at various skeletal sites. *J Bone Min Res*; **6** (suppl. 1): S136.

Neaton JD, Wentworth D, for the multiple risk factor intervention trial Research Group (1992) Serum cholesterol, blood pressure, cigarette smoking and death from coronary artery disease. Overall findings and differences by age for 316 099 white men. *Arch Intern Med*; **152**: 56–64.

Newton-John HF, Morgan DB (1970) The loss of bone with age, osteoporosis, and fractures. *Clin Orthop*; **71**: 229–252.

Phillips S, Fox N, Jacobs J, Wright WE (1988) The direct medical costs of osteoporosis for American women aged 45 and older, 1986. *Bone*; **9**: 271–279.

Royal College of Physicians (1989) *Fractured Neck of Femur. Prevention and Management*. Royal College of Physicians, London.

Urist MR (1973) Orthopedic management of osteoporosis in post menopausal women. *Clin Endocrinol Metab*; **2**: 159–176.

White BL, Fisher WD, Laurin CA (1987) Rate of mortality for elderly patients after fracture of the hip in the 1980s. *J Bone Joint Surg*; **69A**: 1335–1339.

WHO (1994) *Assessment of Osteoporotic Fracture Risk and its Role in Screening for Postmenopausal Osteoporosis*. WHO Technical Report Series, Geneva.

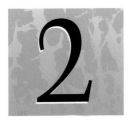

Pathogenesis of osteoporosis and fracture

The risk of osteoporosis depends in part upon skeletal development, the attainment of peak bone mass and in later life on the amount of bone lost. In the mature skeleton osteoporosis arises through the disruption of the processes which normally maintain skeletal balance and turnover which, in turn, affect its competence to withstand the stresses of life. This chapter reviews the manner in which skeletal mass is maintained in adult life, the way in which these processes are perturbed in osteoporosis and the factors which determine the gain and loss of bone throughout life.

Maintenance of bone mass

STRUCTURE AND DISPOSITION OF NORMAL BONE

Types of bone tissue

Broadly, there are two types of bone tissue in the adult, cortical or compact bone, and spongy or cancellous bone. Most bones have an outer cortical casing comprising an outer (periosteal) and inner (cortical endosteal) surface which encloses the cancellous bone and marrow space (Fig. 2.1). In the adult with a total body calcium of approximately 1 kg, 80% of skeletal mass is cortical. The remaining cancellous bone comprises trabecular plates and rods of tissue which interconnect with each other and with the inner aspect of the cortex. The arrangement of bony trabeculae confers a high degree of rigidity to the outer cortical shell and increases markedly the resistance of bone to compressive and tortional forces, even though in most bones it comprises a minor component of bone tissue. The disposition of trabecular plates and rods is orientated predominantly according to lines of stress, and characteristic trabecular patterns are recognized at many sites including the spine, hip and heel.

Bony trabeculae

MATRIX AND MINERAL

Bone comprises an organic matrix, a mineral phase and bone cells. The majority of the matrix is composed of collagen fibres, which account for 90% of skeletal weight in the adult. There are several types of collagen; that of adult bone is type I, which is laid down by

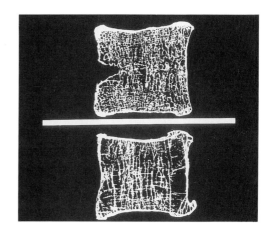

Fig. 2.1 Sagittal section through a lumbar vertebral body showing the casing of cortical bone and the interconnecting lattice of trabeculae. The lower section shows an osteoporotic vertebra. Note the decreased number of trabeculae.

Bone proteins

osteoblasts. Each unit of collagen (tropocollagen) comprises a protein heterotrimer consisting of two α-1 chains and one α-2 chain. Protein synthesis is followed by a number of post-translational modifications, particularly the hydroxylation of proline and lysine. Hydroxyproline and hydroxylysine are not specific to collagen but their release during the metabolism of bone can be utilized as an index of disease activity. Glycosylation and the formation of cross-links with other tropocollagen macromolecules permit their assembly to form collagen fibrils. Evidence of such activity can be measured in serum and urine, and provides further non-invasive indices of skeletal metabolism in the investigation of osteoporosis (see Chapter 5). There are many other important proteins present in bone matrix, including proteoglycans, glycoproteins, osteocalcin and osteonectin, which are incorporated within the collagen matrix during or after its formation. As in the case of collagen products, some of these, particularly osteocalcin, can be used to assess the rate of bone turnover in the evaluation of osteoporosis.

Bone mineral

The mineral phase of bone is mainly calcium, phosphate and carbonate $(10:6:1)$ arranged as crystals predominantly in the form of hydroxyapatite. Mineralization begins with the precipitation of amorphous calcium phosphate and, with time, the mineral phase becomes progressively more crystalline. Crystals of hydroxyapatite are elongated and hexagonal in shape, which conforms closely to the orientation of the collagen fibres. They also contain other ions including sodium, magnesium and fluoride.

BONE SURFACES AND BONE CELLS

Metabolic activity

The metabolic activity of bone is predominantly a surface-based phenomenon, and several different types of bone surface are available in the skeleton, summarized in Table 2.1 (see also Fig. 2.2). The surface available for bone remodelling includes the cancellous and cortical endosteal surface and the vascular channels within bone.

23 / Pathogenesis

This is considerably less than the surface available for mineral exchange, which additionally includes the lacunae and interconnecting canaliculi occupied by osteocytes. Even though cortical bone comprises three-quarters of the total skeletal tissue, the surfaces available in cortical bone are much lower than that of cancellous tissue. Indeed, the surface/volume ratio of cancellous bone is eight- to 10-fold greater than that of cortical bone (see Table 2.1). Since the turnover of bone is a surface-based event, this activity is greater on cancellous than on cortical surfaces. This is one of the reasons why

Table 2.1 Some characteristics of the normal skeleton. (From Kanis, 1991a)

Surfaces (m²)	
Cortical bone	3.5*
Trabecular bone	9*
Osteocyte	90
Lacunar and cannalicular	1200
Mass (g)	
Cortical bone	4000
Trabecular bone	1000
Total skeleton	5000
Surface/mass ratio (cm²/g)*	
Cortical bone	87.5
Trabecular bone	900
Total skeleton	250

* Denotes surfaces available for remodelling.

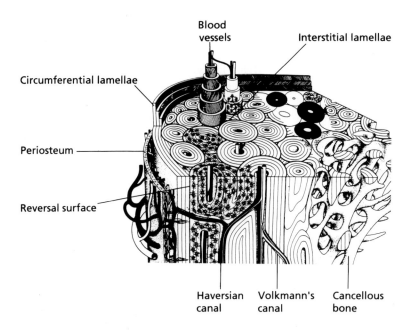

Fig. 2.2 Schematic diagram of diaphyseal cortical bone showing the transverse and longitudinal arrangement of osteons.

osteoporosis is expressed more floridly and earlier at cancellous sites than in cortical bone.

All bone surfaces are covered by cells with distinct morphological and functional features. These include osteoblasts, osteoclasts and osteocytes. The osteoblast is the cell responsible for the synthesis of collagen and other bone proteins. It also has an important role in the subsequent mineralization of the matrix. Once bone is mineralized, some of the osteoblasts are retained on the bone surface and termed 'resting' osteoblasts or bone-lining cells. Osteocytes are osteoblasts which have been trapped within the bone matrix during the process of bone formation. The osteocytes are interconnected to osteoblasts and other osteocytes by fine intercellular projections running within bone canaliculi.

The other major cell type found in bone is the osteoclast. This is a multinucleated cell which is responsible for bone resorption. It preferentially degrades fully mineralized bone by attaching onto a bone surface and secreting acids and lysosomal enzymes into the space provided between its apical surface and the mineralized bone surface. The surface of the osteoclast at this interface is ruffled by cytoplasmic extensions that infiltrate the resorbing bone surface.

REMODELLING OF BONE

In the mature adult, skeletal size is neither increasing nor decreasing. Despite this, bone is continuously being turned over, so that the net activity of bone resorbing cells equals the net activity of bone forming cells. In the adult, this activity is largely accounted for by bone remodelling. Remodelling comprises the process of bone resorption followed by bone formation and provides a mechanism for self repair and adaptation to stress.

The steps involved in the remodelling of bone have been well characterized both in health and in osteoporosis (Fig. 2.3; Parfitt, 1983; Eriksen, 1986). The first visible step of bone remodelling is the focal attraction of osteoclasts to the quiescent bone surface. The factors that determine the site for the focal attraction of a team of osteoclasts are not known, but it is possible that fatigue damage to bone could be a stimulus.

Activation

The attraction of a team of osteoclasts to a locus on the bone surface is termed activation. The term refers to the event and not to the activity of the osteoclasts themselves. Activation frequency describes the frequency with which activation events occur on bone surfaces. In health, an activation occurs every 10 seconds or so, and its frequency will largely determine the number of new remodelling sites present on bone tissue. Both parathyroid hormone (PTH) and thyroid hormones increase activation frequency. Calcitriol also increases the activation frequency but this may be a pharmacological rather than a

Osteoblasts make bone

Osteoclasts resorb bone

Bone turnover

Steps of remodelling

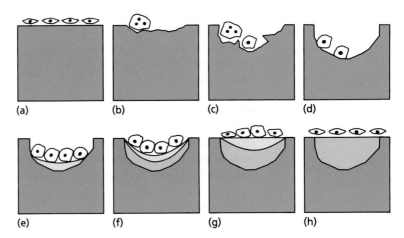

Fig. 2.3 Schematic diagram to show the stages in the remodelling sequence of trabecular bone. (a) Quiescent bone surface. (b) The activation of bone resorption by the focal attraction of osteoclasts. (c) The creation by osteoclasts of a resorption cavity. (d) Smoothing of erosion cavities by mononuclear cells (reversal). (e) The differentiation of osteoblasts within erosion cavities (coupling). (f) The onset of matrix synthesis and mineralization. (g) The completion of matrix synthesis. (h) The completion of the remodelling sequence where the bone surface is covered by lining cells once more.

physiological effect. The gonadal steroids and calcitonins are inhibitors of activation.

Resorption

During the phase of bone resorption the team of osteoclasts cut a depth of up to 20 μm/day on the surface of cancellous bone. During this time, the osteoclast team excavates an erosion cavity to a depth of 40–60 μm over 4–12 days (see Fig. 2.3). Thereafter, the multinucleated cells disappear and are replaced by mononuclear cells which appear to be capable of some resorption and smooth off the resorption cavity. Over the next 7–10 days a layer of cement substance is deposited which is rich in proteoglycans, glycoproteins and acid phosphatase but poor in collagen. This is termed the reversal phase which describes the time interval between the cessation of osteoclast-mediated bone resorption and bone formation (see Fig. 2.3).

Reversal phase

Coupling

Once resorption and reversal are complete, the process termed coupling attracts osteoblasts to the eroded surface which thereafter synthesize an osteoid matrix (see Fig. 2.3). The coupling signal is not known but may be mediated by reversal cells within resorption cavities, the cement substance of the reversal surface, or the exposure of chemotactic proteins within bone matrix such as collagen fragments or transforming growth factors. The amount of new bone formed is also dependent on the number and activity of the osteoblasts present. As in the case of resorption, variations in number and activity can be measured by histological techniques. Osteoblasts form a sheet of cells within the resorption cavity and synthesize layers of osteoid matrix which comprise unmineralized bone tissue and other matrix proteins. Matrix synthesis is rapid during the initiation of the formation phase. The newly formed osteoid has a lamellated arrangement of collagen due to changes in the orientation of collagen bundles which are well visualized under polarized light. In cancellous bone the lamellae are usually parallel to the trabeculae.

Formation

Mineralization
A few days after the onset of matrix formation by osteoblasts, the newly formed osteoid undergoes mineralization (Eriksen, 1986). The delay between the onset of matrix synthesis and the start of mineralization accounts for the appearance of osteoid in normal bone, during which maturation of osteoid occurs as well as the incorporation of other bone proteins. The first steps in calcification are thought to take place in or around small membrane-bound vesicles, rich in alkaline phosphatase, an enzyme which has been known for many years to be associated with calcification. This ectoenzyme is shedded from the osteoblast into the extracellular fluid and the measurement of its activity in serum provides one of the biochemical indices of skeletal metabolism widely used in clinical practice. Osteocalcin (bone gla protein) is another of several bone proteins produced exclusively by osteoblasts and is also measured in serum. Its function is not certain but it may be important for the adsorption of mineral onto bone matrix. Mineralization can be detected by stains such as toluidine blue or on ultraviolet fluorescence by prelabelling bone with tetracyclines. When osteoblast synthesis of matrix is complete, the morphology of the osteoblast changes, and during mineralization they become elongated. When mineralization is accomplished, the resting osteoblasts become flattened and complete the remodelling sequence.

Alkaline phosphatase

Osteocalcin

The sequence of activation, resorption, reversal, formation and mineralization occurs normally on the minority of the bone surface; at any one time 90% or so of available surfaces are inert. A similar sequence of events occurs in cortical bone (Fig. 2.4). The moiety of bone formed, termed a bone structural unit (BSU) takes several months to be synthesized and mineralized. In contrast, the process of osteoclastic bone resorption is complete within days. This explains why formation surfaces on bone are more abundant than resorption surfaces. Since bone formation rates and the surface extent of formation can be measured, the time period of all events on bone surfaces can be calculated from bone biopsies.

Bone structural unit

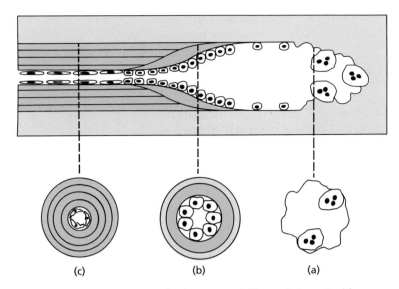

Fig. 2.4 Schematic diagram of a bone remodelling unit in cortical bone. Osteoclasts tunnel in the long axis of the cortex to create a cutting cone (a). The erosion cavity is smoothed off during the reversal phase. Thereafter, osteoblasts synthesize an osteoid matrix in the form of concentric lamellae (b) which infill the erosion cavity (c) leaving a new Haversian canal. Note that unlike trabecular bone the resorption cavity cannot be overfilled. (From Kanis, 1991a.)

BRUs AND BSUs

The remodelling sequence in both cancellous and cortical bone involves an organized and focal series of cellular events which are termed bone remodelling units (BRUs). The completion of activity of a BRU results in the creation of a BSU. In the case of cortical bone the BSU is a secondary osteon or Haversian system and cylindrical in shape. In cancellous bone the BSU is flat, $40-60\,\mu m$ thick with an area of $0.5-1\,mm^2$. The thickness of a completed BSU is relatively constant and termed the wall thickness. It is reduced in some forms of osteoporosis denoting a decrease in the amount of bone formed within each resorption cavity. Of 35 million BSUs in skeletal tissue, approximately 40% are in cancellous bone (Parfitt, 1983).

Bone remodelling and bone loss in osteoporosis

Osteoporosis is often considered to be a type of bone atrophy. Whereas this may describe the end-result, the events which occur in bone at and after the menopause include a generalized increase in its activity. Studies in mammals indicate a two- to threefold increase in cellular activity of bone surfaces due to an increase in activation frequency which occurs after oestrogen deficiency. No studies of the time course of histological events have been done in postmenopausal

Cellular activity

osteoporosis, but an indication of this comes from studies of the indirect indices of skeletal turnover following oophorectomy or a natural menopause. After oophorectomy, the earliest event is an increase in the urinary excretion of hydroxyproline due to an increase in activation and the subsequent increase in bone resorption. This is followed by a later increase in bone formation, as judged by the activity of alkaline phosphatase or serum osteocalcin (Stepan et al., 1987). This pattern of response is consistent with a primary increase in bone resorption followed by a coupled increment in bone formation, so that all the elements of turnover are increased.

Increased turnover

The number of osteoclasts in osteoporosis is increased on average by two- to threefold. Whereas this is associated with an increase in the activation frequency of bone remodelling, it is also likely that the numbers of osteoclasts that differentiate within each resorption bay are also increased in the early postmenopause. The net effect is that, not only is the extent of resorption increased, but so too is the depth of the resorption cavity. An increase in the depth of erosion, if sufficient, may transect trabecular elements, and trabecular plate perforation is a conspicuous feature of postmenopausal osteoporosis or secondary hypogonadism in the male (Parfitt et al., 1983). A similar process occurs following prolonged immobilization and hyperparathyroidism, but in corticosteroid-induced osteoporosis trabecular thinning occurs with little loss of trabecular numbers (Aaron et al., 1989).

New bone formation

As in normal bone remodelling, resorption by osteoclasts is followed by new bone formation. The numbers of osteoblasts are increased to match the increase in the resorption surface, but after the menopause a decrease in mineral apposition rate is found and the performance of individual osteoblasts is less than normal (Parfitt et al., 1981). The manner in which oestrogens affect osteoblast performance is not known. It may be a direct effect, since there is evidence that osteoblasts have oestrogen receptors.

Oestrogen receptors

When remodelling is complete the thickness of the structural unit is termed the wall thickness. Wall thickness decreases with age in women (Fig. 2.5), and is more markedly decreased in corticosteroid-induced osteoporosis, during immobilization and in myelomatosis, indicating that each erosion cavity is infilled with a smaller than normal volume of bone. Thus, even where the depth of erosion is normal, each remodelling sequence is associated with a small but finite deficit in bone. If the depth of erosion is also increased, bone loss is accentuated. Where the depth of erosion is shallow, little loss of bone may occur.

Remodelling imbalance

The amount of osteoid present in osteoporotic bone is greater than that seen in healthy bone. This does not necessarily imply the presence of osteomalacia, which is a defect in the mineralization process. Accelerated bone turnover increases the frequency of all events on bone surfaces including the surface extent of osteoid. Osteomalacia

Osteomalacia

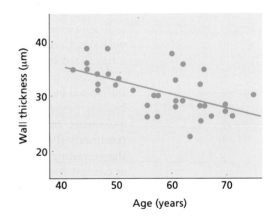

Fig. 2.5 Wall thickness according to age in healthy postmenopausal women. $P < 0.01$. (Data from Recker *et al.*, 1988.)

is more common in the elderly and, when present, may complicate osteoporosis and contribute to skeletal fragility. The finding of an increase in osteoid seam width and more than five osteoid lamellae should alert one to the possibility of coexisting osteomalacia. It is characterized by thick osteoid seams due to a delay or absence in the mineralization of bone.

MECHANISMS OF BONE LOSS

Increased bone turnover

In postmenopausal osteoporosis or in response to immobilization, the increase in bone turnover has several effects on bone mineral mass. The process of bone remodelling implies a net deficit of bone (until resorption cavities are completely infilled) so that the skeletal volume missing at any one time will increase proportionately according to the number of functional BRUs (Fig. 2.6). This skeletal deficit

Resorption space

is termed the resorption space and is equivalent to 7.6 g of calcium or 0.76% of total body calcium.

A further consequence of increased skeletal remodelling relates to the decreased turnover time of the skeleton. An increase in mineral density occurs for 1 or 2 years after the apparent completion of the

Fig. 2.6 Effect of bone turnover on bone and calcium balance. The upper panel depicts normal bone remodelling activity occurring on 15% of the trabecular surface. The resorption space occupies 2% of the bone volume and a somewhat smaller amount (1.5%) is occupied by osteoid accounting for 3.5% of the bone volume. When turnover is increased fivefold (without affecting the balance between formation and resorption) the resorption space and osteoid space increase to 17.5%. In addition, new bone formed at each site is not completely mineralized, increasing the mineral deficit to 19% of trabecular density.

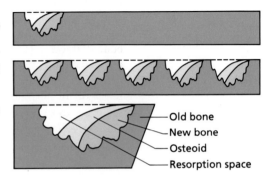

remodelling unit. If bone turnover is accelerated, a proportionately greater amount of bone volume is occupied by young rather than by old BSUs. Consequently, the proportion of immature and incompletely mineralized bone will increase.

For these reasons, the mineral content of bone may be profoundly influenced by changes in bone turnover alone. A fivefold increase in bone turnover would produce a negative calcium balance of 30 g or a decrease in total body bone volume of 3% under steady-state conditions (Parfitt, 1983). The change in bone volume depends on the prevailing rate of bone turnover, and is greater at cancellous than at cortical sites. In the trabecular bone of the ilium, the remodelling space is approximately 5% of the bone volume. Consequently, a fivefold increase in turnover would decrease the actual bone volume by 20% and the mineral content by nearly double (see Fig. 2.6). The effects at cortical sites will be less. The rate of change of bone mass is not linear. It is initially rapid and thereafter declines and takes several years to be complete. It accounts in some measure for the accelerated losses which occur at the time of the menopause or after immobilization. Losses due to high turnover alone are theoretically reversible if bone turnover is decreased. This is not always true since accelerated turnover may itself damage the structural integrity of cancellous bone (discussed below).

REMODELLING AND FOCAL SKELETAL BALANCE

It is useful to draw a distinction between skeletal balance and the coupling of bone formation to bone resorption. Uncoupling implies the dissociation of these two processes; either the creation of resorption cavities without subsequent attraction of osteoblasts, as is sometimes seen in neoplasia, or conversely, the deposition of new bone at sites other than sites of previous resorption. The latter occurs conspicuously in various tumours, such as prostatic bone disease, or in osteoporosis following treatment with fluoride. In the case of untreated post-menopausal osteoporosis there is no direct evidence for uncoupled bone resorption even in the presence of marked osteoporosis.

Over and above the effects of an increase in bone turnover alone on bone mass, subsequent steady-state changes in bone volume are due to focal imbalances at remodelling sites, related in turn to changes in the functional capacity or numbers of osteoblasts and osteoclasts involved in the BRU. Since wall thickness (the depth of BSUs on bone surfaces after the completion of bone formation) is markedly decreased in osteoporosis (see Fig. 2.5), the balance between the amount formed and that resorbed at each remodelling site is tipped

in favour of net bone resorption at this site. If at each remodelling sequence there is a focal imbalance, then the rate of change of bone volume will depend on the activation frequency. If the rate of bone turnover is increased threefold then the rate of change of bone tissue volume is trebled (Fig. 2.7).

31 / Pathogenesis

Fig. 2.7 Schematic representation of a trabecular bone surface to illustrate the effect of balance and remodelling on bone loss. (a) Shows the infilling of a resorption cavity with an equal volume of new bone. (b) Shows less bone deposited at a site of previous resorption. If bone turnover is increased without altering this balance (c), the rate of trabecular bone loss will increase in proportion to the increment in bone turnover.

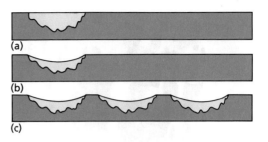

ARCHITECTURAL ABNORMALITIES OF TRABECULAR BONE

The continual imbalance between formation and resorption in osteoporosis might be expected to result in a progressive decrease in the width of trabecular bone elements. This occurs in some forms of osteoporosis, but in postmenopausal osteoporosis and after immobil-

Loss of trabecular numbers

ization there is a marked loss of trabecular numbers (Parfitt *et al.*, 1983; Parfitt, 1987). Trabecular numbers are decreased by 45% in postmenopausal osteoporosis, whereas in corticosteroid-induced osteoporosis, numbers are only decreased by 10% (Aaron *et al.*, 1989) but the width of remaining trabeculae is markedly decreased. The lack of evidence for trabecular thinning in postmenopausal osteoporosis indicates that the loss of trabeculae arise as a result of the generation of deep resorption cavities which transect the trabecular structures. The remaining trabeculae hypertrophy in response to the increased load. It is also probable that where a trabecular rod is transected, the decreased stress in the remnant structure results in further resorption so that the process becomes accentuated, and the potential surface on which to attract osteoblasts for new matrix synthesis is even less.

Cancellous bone strength

The destruction of cross-bracing trabecular elements has marked implications for the strength of cancellous bone (Vesterby *et al.*, 1991). The resistance of a cross-braced rod to bending is proportional to the square of the distance between the bracing structures, so that trabecular losses weaken the bone tissue out of proportion to the amount lost. A further consequence of the destruction of trabecular elements is that treatments which exploit the remodelling sequence can only be effective where pre-existing bone surfaces are found. This means that many treatments are likely to thicken remnant structures rather than restore the connectivity of bone (see Chapter 7).

FATIGUE DAMAGE

Repeated stress

Like all solid structures, bone undergoes damage from repeated stresses, but unlike inert materials, it can self-repair. If the remodelling activity of bone is impaired, this can give rise to stress fractures. In osteoporosis there is less bone so that strains induced by activity are greater. In addition, the turnover of bone may decrease once the

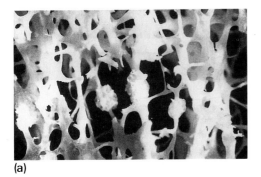
(a)

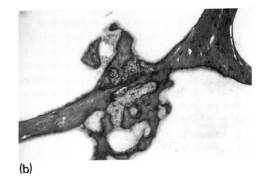
(b)

Fig. 2.8 (a) Microphotograph to show the presence of callus formation arising from microfractures in cancellous bone of the femoral neck. (From Todd *et al.*, 1972.) Note that they are more evident on weight bearing (vertical) trabeculae. Note also the preferential decrease in width of horizontal trabeculae. (b) Shows a histological section through a microfracture and the surrounding callus. (Courtesy of Dr J. Aaron.)

process of trabecular loss is complete, so that the turnover of remaining bone is low, and the bone is stiffer. Increased numbers of microfractures are found with age (Fig. 2.8; Todd *et al.*, 1972; Vernon-Roberts & Pirie, 1973) and more frequently in osteoporotic bone.

Microfractures heal initially by woven rather than lamellar bone formation in much the same way as seen in normal fracture repair (see Fig. 2.8). Although microcallus can calcify in the same way as callus, its disorganized nature means that it preferentially takes up bone-seeking agents such as fluorides which complicate the treatment of osteoporosis (see Chapter 8).

Microfractures

CORTICAL BONE LOSS

Whereas longitudinal growth ceases in early adult life, net periosteal apposition continues throughout life so that the width of several tubular bones and, indeed, the vertebral bodies increase with age (Garn, 1970; Mosekilde & Mosekilde, 1990). Increased width of bones occurs through remodelling activity rather than by continuous apposition of bone (modelling). There is no evidence that this progressive increase in width is perturbed in osteoporosis, though the attainment of maximal width is impaired in primary gonadal insufficiency. The increase in circumference of long bones is more than offset by endocortical losses so that the width of the cortex decreases with age, a phenomenon which is more marked in patients who sustain osteoporotic fractures.

Bone width

Cortical thickness

The decrease in cortical thickness that occurs with aging is also mediated by remodelling, but is clearly dependent on gonadal status. It is of interest that different bone-active drugs have different effects at the different endosteal surfaces. These include the vitamin Ds and the anabolic and gonadal steroids. For example, the anabolic steroids appear to affect endocortical sites differently from trabecular bone (see Chapter 8). In contrast, the use of vitamin D analogues does not prevent endocortical losses, but may decrease bone losses at cancellous sites. This suggests that the processes governing endocortical turnover might differ from those governing trabecular bone. Both clearly differ from the factors influencing turnover at the periosteum.

TYPES OF OSTEOPOROSIS

Two types

It has been suggested that osteoporosis can be divided into two types according to the turnover of bone (high and low turnover osteoporosis). Histological findings are heterogeneous in women with

High and low turnover

osteoporosis. For this reason, the terms high and low turnover osteoporosis are commonly used (Meunier *et al.*, 1981; Whyte *et al.*, 1982), but the histological findings probably reflect a continuum rather than two disorders. A component of heterogeneity could be due to secondary hyperparathyroidism related to aging or vitamin D deficiency.

A second approach to the classification of osteoporosis is based on the differences between cortical and cancellous bone volume. For

Cortical and cancellous

example, cancellous bone volume is lower in patients with trochanteric than cervical fractures, but differences in cortical width are less evident (Lips *et al.*, 1982).

Type I and type II

A third classification of osteoporosis that has been proposed is to divide this into type I and type II on the basis of clinical characteristics. The notion is that type I accounts for cancellous fractures such as vertebral crush fracture, and that type II gives rise predominantly to cortical fractures such as those at the hip. Patients with hip fracture appear to have narrower cortical margins than patients with vertebral fracture, whereas patients with vertebral fracture have lower cancellous bone volumes than hip fracture patients (Johnston *et al.*, 1985).

Irrespective of the classification proposed, there is evidence for heterogeneity of bone mass in patients with osteoporosis. This includes evidence that the amount of bone present in patients with specific osteoporotic fractures is lower at that site than in patients with fractures elsewhere (see Chapter 3). Whereas the notion of two different types of bone loss is a widely prevalent view, the heterogeneity of bone volume may reflect differences in peak bone mass rather than differences in skeletal losses. Indeed, as reviewed later in this chapter, bone capital at maturity is the major determinant of bone mass in most individuals, at least up to the age of 75 years.

Peak bone mass

The amount of bone mineral present in the skeleton is a function of the amount that is gained during the phase of skeletal development and maturation, and that which is lost. It is convenient therefore to consider the determinants of bone gain separately from the determinants of bone loss.

Bone gain

Skeletal growth and development continues over several decades. Skeletal calcification begins before birth, particularly during the third trimester. At birth, total body calcium is about 25 g and increases to 1000 g or more at skeletal maturity. Growth is most prominent in the first few years after birth and thereafter at the adolescent growth spurt. This is one reason why some believe that nutritional factors are particularly important at these periods for skeletal development. At these times the demands for calcium are particularly high but are less marked than might be suggested by the increase in height (Parfitt, 1983). This is because remodelling activity also increases, which in turn increases cortical porosity and the resorption space. Thus, bone mineral content increases less than expected for the increase in skeletal size. In late adolescence bone remodelling decreases in parallel with longitudinal growth and bone mineral density increases.

The phase between the cessation of longitudinal skeletal growth and the attainment of peak bone mineral or mass has been termed
Consolidation
consolidation. This comprises the expected increases in bone mineral related to a decrease in bone turnover and changes in cortical width. The extent and the duration of consolidation are not well documented by longitudinal studies. Recent studies suggest that consolidation continues until the third decade of life (Recker *et al.*, 1992), but other longitudinal studies at sites of cancellous bone have not shown increases over this age range (Bonjour *et al.* 1991) and population studies indicate little increase in cortical bone mass between the ages of 20 and 35 years (Garn, 1970). Consolidation occurs more rapidly at some sites than at others and varies between sexes so that in adulthood, skeletal mass is 10–50% higher in men than in women depending on the skeletal site measured. The differences between sexes is more marked at cortical and appendicular sites.

Determinants of peak bone mass

Many factors have been suggested to influence the attainment of peak skeletal mass (Table 2A).

It is important to recognize, however, that a small skeleton does not necessarily equate with an increased risk of fracture in later life. Thus, factors which determine skeletal size are not necessarily factors which determine skeletal fragility.

RACIAL AND GENETIC FACTORS

A number of studies suggest an important genetic component in the determination of peak bone mass and in some instances the

Table 2A Factors that have been thought to be determinants of peak skeletal mass

Genetic Racial (risk lower in black people) Familial history (−)
Nutritional Calcium (±) Vitamin D (+) Malnutrition (−)
Exercise Daily physical activity (+) Immobilization (−) Space flight (−)
Other environmental factors Smoking (−)
Hormonal factors Delayed puberty (−) Primary gonadal insufficiency (−) Secondary gonadal failure (−) Use of oral contraceptives (±) Multiparity (±) Lactation (±) Premenstrual tension (−)

+ Denotes a protective factor, − a risk and ± denotes that the evidence for both exists.

susceptibility to later fractures. The evidence is provided from several different types of investigation:
1 the study of bone mineral content or fracture rates in different races;
2 twin studies comparing bone mineral in monozygotic and dizygotic twins;
3 the study of bone mineral content in families.

There are important racial differences in bone density. A good example is black people who have a higher bone density even when adjusted for body weight and height. They also have a lower incidence of osteoporotic fractures (Melton, 1991). Differences in bone vertebral density become apparent in the late stage of puberty but differences in cortical bone mass are present throughout childhood. Differences in bone mass alone may not fully explain the differences in fracture risk. For example, the frequency of falling is less in black people than among whites (Cummings & Nevitt, 1989). Studies of twins have shown less differences in bone mass between monozygotic than dizygotic twins. With one exception (Moller *et al.*, 1978) these studies have been based on absorptiometric techniques, so that it is difficult to distinguish the relative components of skeletal size and true

Differences in bone mass

differences in bone density (see Chapter 5). Indeed, the heritability of height is probably as great as that reported for apparent density. With advancing age, these differences are less apparent, suggesting that environmental factors assume a greater importance. In youth, 50% or so of the variance in bone density may be due to genetic factors, depending on the site of measurement and the assumptions made. It is difficult, however, to distinguish environmental from genetic factors. Such studies provide, therefore, a maximal estimate of heritability. Recent studies suggest that approximately 50% of the apparent heritability may be associated with variations in the vitamin D receptor gene.

Bone mass is also lower in daughters of osteoporotic patients, but the effect is small and not invariably found. Several types of osteoporosis have very clear patterns of inheritance; for example, osteogenesis imperfecta. These are described in Chapter 4. Patients with mild osteogenesis imperfecta may present for the first time in adulthood, particularly women after the menopause. Unless this is recognized, it increases the apparent heritability of osteoporosis. For these reasons environmental factors may have been underestimated. A good example is provided by the low bone mass of the Japanese which is higher in Japanese immigrants to the United States, and is even higher in Americans of Japanese descent (Nomura et al., 1989).

GONADAL STATUS

The marked difference in fracture risk between men and women is likely to relate in part to the differences in peak bone mass between men and women.

Delayed puberty

A constitutional delay in puberty decreases the ultimate height of individuals. Spinal growth is more markedly impaired compared to that of the long bones, and final bone mineral density is decreased in men and women. Normal variations in the age of puberty may contribute to bone density and fracture risk, since an early menarche is associated with a significant decrease in fracture risk and higher bone mineral density (BMD).

Factors known to delay menarche are the many causes of malnutrition (critical weight achieved at a later age), and living at high altitude. Twins tend to have a later menarche. Physical exercise may also delay menarche. For example, the menarcheal age of athletes who begin training before the age of menarche was 2 years later than the age of athletes who began training after menarche (Frisch et al., 1981) suggesting that training rather than pre-selection was the more important factor. These determinants of age of menarche may be related to changes in total body composition, particularly in fat mass, that occur before menarche, and premenarcheal changes in pituitary gonadotrophin activity, ovarian and adrenal function.

Primary and secondary gonadal failure

Skeletal mass

Turner's syndrome and Klinefelter's syndrome are both associated with a decrease in bone mass and an increased risk of osteoporotic fractures in later life. Cortical width is decreased before puberty, suggesting that other genetic factors may also contribute to decreased skeletal mass. Notwithstanding, all causes of gonadal failure cause loss of skeletal mass, so that intermittent gonadal failure before the menopause may account for a low bone mineral density in later life. Examples include anorexia nervosa, exercise-induced gonadal failure, and prolactinoma where this induces gonadal changes. The relative importance of oestrogen deficiency compared with environmental factors such as nutrition and exercise is demonstrated in exercise-induced gonadal failure, where bone loss occurs despite adequate nutrition and abundant exercise (Drinkwater et al., 1984).

Breast feeding

More subtle alterations in gonadal status might alter adult bone mass. These include parity and lactation which have been reported (inconsistently) as protective factors. Retrospective surveys have variously shown breast feeding to be associated with increased or decreased (BMD). There are relatively few prospective studies, but these suggest that bone mineral content (BMC) is decreased during lactation (Hayslip et al., 1989) and may be reversible (Sowers et al., 1993).

Parity

The conclusions concerning the effect of parity on bone mass are equally disparate when population studies are examined. Prospective studies show no change in total body calcium during pregnancy but decreases in bone density at the hip and forearm have been measured by dual photon absorptiometry (Drinkwater & Chesnut, 1991). In this study tibial bone mass increased. The changes were small, however, and may have been in part artefactual due to changes in body composition.

Oral contraceptives

Similarly, the use of oral contraceptives is reported to be associated with a higher lumbar BMC at maturity than in women who do not use oral contraceptives (Recker et al., 1992). Others have shown no effect at skeletal maturity. There is a problem in ascribing causality from all these population studies; for example, women who elect to breastfeed, use contraceptives or get pregnant differ in many other cultural ways which might not be immediately obvious.

NUTRITIONAL FACTORS

Dietary effect on bone mass

Many nutritional factors have been invoked as important for the attainment or maintenance of bone mass, including the dietary intake of protein, sodium, tea, coffee and alcohol. Some of these are reviewed elsewhere (see Chapter 4) since they are regarded by some as causes of osteoporosis. In addition the contribution of these factors to peak bone mass, bone loss and fracture risk is uncertain. By far the greatest attention has focused on the effect of calcium on peak BMD.

Calcium

It is evident that without calcium there would be no skeleton – or at least it would not be mineralized. The question is not therefore whether calcium is important, but rather how much calcium is required. The recommended daily allowance of calcium for healthy women varies from country to country, and ranges from 400 to 1500 mg daily (Trusswell *et al.*, 1983). Higher intakes are commonly recommended in adolescence and pregnancy.

How much required?

It is argued that most of the world's population consume less than 500 mg daily, and that there is little convincing evidence that those countries with lower dietary intakes are disadvantaged in regard to bone mineral at maturity (Kanis & Passmore, 1989; Kanis, 1991b). This view has been vigorously challenged by Nordin & Heaney (1990) who defend a recommended daily allowance (RDA) of 1000 mg in young healthy adults, largely on the basis of the same evidence reviewed by ourselves. It is important therefore to examine the foundations on which these different recommendations are based.

Recommended daily allowance

It is first relevant to recall two aspects of bone remodelling in the adult which are of importance in thinking about the requirements for calcium. Firstly, the accretion of calcium into bone occurs after matrix production and not before (see Chapter 1). Thus, the skeletal demands for calcium are governed by the rate of matrix synthesis rather than the other way round. If the skeletal demands for calcium are not met, then hypocalcaemia and defective mineralization of bone will follow as has been shown in mammals. The question arises whether low dietary intakes of calcium might decrease bone matrix synthesis in humans, but most evidence suggests that calcium supplementation decreases rather than increases the rate of turnover of bone. This suggests that under normal conditions the skeletal requirements for calcium are governed by the rate of matrix synthesis rather than by the availability of calcium.

Rate of matrix synthesis governs demand for calcium

Secondly, changes in the dietary intake of calcium are capable of inducing changes in the rate of bone turnover. In the healthy adult who has an inadequate dietary intake of calcium, the rate of bone turnover is increased due to an increase in the activation frequency with the expected consequences on skeletal density (see Chapter 1). Conversely, when presented with high calcium challenges bone remodelling is decreased. A great deal of circumstantial evidence suggests that the mechanism for this relates to hormonal changes in calcium metabolism. Thus, during calcium depletion serum calcium tends to fall, which stimulates the secretion of PTH and the synthesis of calcitriol (see Chapter 3), which in turn increases the activation of bone remodelling and induces a small but finite decrease in bone mass.

Changes in calcium intake affect rate of turnover

Prospective controlled studies to show whether an increase in calcium intake increases peak bone mass independently of energy intake in children are equivocal, and have generally shown no effect on growth. The most recent study examining this issue showed that the addition of a calcium load during growth had very small effects on skeletal mass, entirely explicable by differences in the rate of bone remodelling (Johnston *et al.*, 1992). Nor are there randomized studies available to determine whether an increased calcium intake has any significant effect on skeletal consolidation or subsequent risk of fracture after longitudinal growth has ceased.

A variety of epidemiological studies show an association between the lifetime intake of calcium and either bone density or the risk of fracture in women. On the other hand, it should be recognized that many studies show no such association over a range of dietary intakes. A starting point in explaining the different findings is related to other nutritional differences between populations. The most cited and complete information available is that from Matkovic *et al.* (1979) showing a relationship between calcium intake, bone mass and fracture from two communities in the former Yugoslavia. One community had a substantially higher calcium intake and the greater bone mass and fewer femoral fractures. Although the calcium intake was higher, so too was the energy intake (Table 2.2), but the mean body weight in the two communities was identical. Lower energy intake in populations with similar body weight indicates less physical activity, and diminished activity is a well-recognized factor affecting

Energy intake

Table 2.2 Nutritional and energy intake (mean ± SD) in women from two communities (A and B) in the former Yugoslavia (100 for each group). Note the significantly higher energy intake in women taking the higher calcium diets despite the similarity in body weight. (Data from Matkovic *et al.*, 1979)

	A High dietary calcium	B Low dietary calcium	A/B	$P<$
Calcium				
(mg/day)	876 ± 280	395 ± 276	2.22	0.001
Protein				
(g/day)	84.4 ± 19.5	56.9 ± 16.5	1.48	0.001
(kcal/day)	346 ± 80	233 ± 68	1.48	0.001
Fat				
(g/day)	92.6 ± 23.5	59.8 ± 21.2	1.55	0.001
(kcal/day)	861 ± 219	556 ± 197	1.55	0.001
Carbohydrate				
(g/day)	327 ± 71	345 ± 80	0.95	NS
(kcal/day)	1341 ± 291	1415 ± 328	0.95	NS
Body weight				
(kg)	68.8 ± 6.0	68.8 ± 6.0	1.00	NS
Total energy				
(kcal/day)	2548 ± 539	2204 ± 389	1.02	0.02
Waking energy expenditure				
(kcal/day)	2086 ± 539	1742 ± 389	1.20	0.02

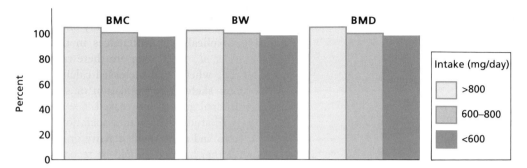

Fig. 2.9 Bone mineral content (BMC), bone width (BW) and apparent bone mineral density (BMD) at the distal radius in elderly American women divided according to current intake of calcium. Values were adjusted for age, energy, protein and phosphorus intake. (From Anderson & Tylavsky, 1984.)

skeletal mass. The data suggest that energy expenditure was 20% greater in the community with the hgher dietary intake of calcium. This suggests that differences in fracture rates may have been due to differences in habitual exercise.

Indeed, other studies have taken activity or energy expenditure into account and shown a significant and independent relationship between calcium intake and bone density. The differences in skeletal mass between high and low intakes of calcium were trivial however, and readily accounted for by differences in the reversible calcium space (Fig. 2.9). These considerations suggest that requirements for calcium cannot be made on the basis of the presently available epidemiological evidence. Studies of metabolic balance are thus the cornerstone for any justification of the RDA.

The computation of the recommended daily allowance in young healthy adults comes from the studies examining the relationship of skeletal or calcium balance to calcium intake. Women on low calcium diets are in negative calcium balance and conversely, women who consume greater amounts are in positive balance (Heaney *et al.*, 1977). It has been argued on this basis that the availability of calcium in many women is inadequate to satisfy the skeletal demands for calcium and, furthermore, that osteoporosis is therefore due to calcium deficiency. The requirement for calcium is estimated from the relationship between intake and balance. The intercept of the regression suggests that the requirements in women before the menopause are in the order of 1 g daily, and are even greater in postmenopausal women. Similar arguments have been put forward concerning the requirements in adolescents (Fig. 2.10).

The calculation of dietary requirements from balance studies is, however, a statistical artefact, and this type of evidence should no longer be used to promote the view that large dietary intakes of calcium are required to maintain skeletal health (Kanis, 1991b). The correlation between dietary intake and balance is an inevitable conse-

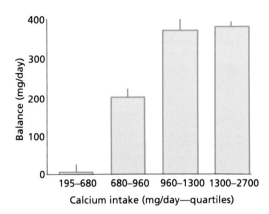

Fig. 2.10 Relationship between dietary intake of calcium and the metabolic balance for calcium in adolescents. Note the apparent dose response suggesting maximal benefits from intakes of 1000 mg or more. (From Matkovic, 1991.)

quence of plotting two dependent variables. The artefact arises because calcium intake is a measurement used in both sides of the equation (balance = intake − excretion).

Several further arguments that are even less convincing have been pursued to defend a RDA of 1000 mg or more. The least satisfactory is the view that it is wise to err on the side of exuberance since calcium does no harm, and may do good. If the premise were accepted that a gram of calcium was essential for skeletal health, the vast majority of the world's population would be calcium deficient, and therefore at a disadvantage. This not only provokes anxiety, but, if untrue, damages the credibility of nutritionists and the medical profession. Moreover, the resource implications for world health are enormous. A more honest approach would be to admit that we do not yet know the necessary requirement, but that there is no good evidence to suggest that variations in dietary intake of calcium are prejudicial for skeletal health in young individuals who take a reasonably balanced diet. Different considerations apply to the use of calcium in later life (see Chapter 7).

Vitamin D

The recommended daily allowance is 400 IU for children and adults in most countries, and is the same as the dose required to prevent

Osteomalacia

the development of osteomalacia. Prolonged vitamin D deficiency in childhood decreases stature and peak bone mass, but the relationship of this to osteoporotic fracture risk in later life is not known. Delayed puberty due to prolonged vitamin D deficiency is likely to decrease bone mass in relation to the height attained.

Fluoride

Fluorosis

Fluoride in the water may give rise to fluorosis, characterized by increases in bone density (see Chapter 9). Several studies have compared fracture rates or differences in bone mineral measurements between communities with a high or low fluoride concentration in the water supply and have concluded that fluoridation of water to

1 ppm was beneficial, as judged by differences in hip fracture rate. Other studies have not reached the same conclusion (Melton, 1990), suggesting that reasons other than fluoridation are likely to explain the differences in fracture rates.

EXERCISE AND PHYSICAL ACTIVITY

Although physical activity is an important determinant of peak bone mass it is important to distinguish between different forms of physical activity, such as weight bearing from non-weight bearing (perhaps better defined as movement), occupational from recreational, and jogging from isometric exercises, since they have different effects.

Many studies have shown a relationship between bone mass and activity in population studies. In addition, women with osteoporotic fractures have a lower muscle mass and strength than age-matched controls. Population studies also show close correlations between bone mass and muscle weight, and vigorous athletic activity and bone mass. In some instances the increases in BMD may be artefactual due to an increase in lean body mass, a decrease in fat mass, or both, which affects the accuracy of the measurements made.

Nearly all community based epidemiological data suggest that lack of physical activity is a risk factor for osteoporotic fracture. Most studies are retrospective in nature, and it is difficult to dissociate the effects of exercise in youth from those in later life, and other confounding factors.

The incidence of various types of osteoporotic fractures has increased in many countries and, after accounting for age and gender, the risk of hip fracture doubled in the United Kingdom over the 30-year interval between the 1950s and 1980s (Boyce & Vessey, 1985). Age-adjusted rates have similarly increased in other European countries and Hong Kong, but appear to have levelled off in the northern United States (Melton, 1993). A decrease in physical exercise is a plausible explanation for the secular trend. In the United Kingdom, food consumption has declined but body mass has stayed the same (Kanis & Passmore, 1989). This indicates that energy expenditure and habitual activity have progressively decreased.

Few studies have examined whether differences in energy expenditure might account for differences in peak bone mass between communities. Differences in the incidence of hip fracture between rural and mountainous communities are consistent with a trophic effect of exercise, and may be explained by differences in bone mass (Gardsell *et al.*, 1991). As mentioned, the differences in bone mass and hip fracture risk in two communities from the former Yugoslavia (Matkovic *et al.*, 1979) are more likely to be related to differences in energy expenditure than to differences in calcium nutrition.

A problem with all these studies relating activity to bone mass or to fracture is that the more robust members of the community might be more inclined to undertake a physical lifestyle, so that self-

43 / Pathogenesis

selection may be a considerable source of bias. The effects of exercise can best be studied prospectively, either following exercise regimens or following studies of immobilization.

Skeletal loading

The best evidence for an important effect of skeletal loading comes from animal experiments which show the consistent dependence of load bearing on skeletal mass (Rubin & Lanyon, 1985). Indeed the effects of loading are so marked that bone loading has been considered to be the primary determinant of bone mass. Viewed in this way the general shape of bone is genetically determined, but bone mass and the disposition of skeletal architecture determines the degree of response to load bearing. Similarly, osteoporosis represents a failure of

Mechanostat

the mechanism which Frost (1992) has referred to as the mechanostat, which is set at different levels by hormonal or dietary factors. In experimental studies, disuse results in an increase in activation frequency and a focal imbalance in favour of resorption, and this is prevented by repetitive strains (Rubin & Lanyon, 1985). The response appears to depend upon the strain induced, and in animals remarkably few periods of dynamic strain are required to exert a maximal effect.

There is some evidence that exercise regimens involving weight-bearing activities may increase skeletal mass in young healthy adults (see Chapter 6), but the effects are relatively small compared to what

Physical stress

might have been predicted from epidemiological data. In agreement with animal studies, more marked effects are noted on bone mass by altering the manner in which stress is applied to the skeleton (Fig. 2.11). There are no randomized prospective data to assess whether an increase in levels of exercise affect skeletal mass at maturity, and this would be a very difficult study to undertake. In contrast, there are a plethora of prospective studies which indicate that lack of physical

Disposition of bone architecture

activity results in bone loss (see Chapter 4).

A more important response to exercise may be in the disposition

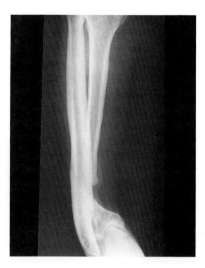

Fig. 2.11 Hypertrophy of the fibula in a man subjected to tibial osteotomy as a child. (Courtesy of J. Chalmers.)

of bone architecture. Football (soccer) players are prone to stress fractures at the beginning of the season rather than a month or so after training. Similarly, army recruits classically sustain stress fractures during the early induction period rather than later.

> It seems likely that the rapid increase in the resistance to stress damage is related to remodelling activity which changes the disposition of the internal trabecular architecture, rather than to the small changes in bone mass that might be induced over such periods.

Patterns and determinants of bone loss

Components of bone loss

It is widely believed that there are several distinct components of the bone loss that occurs with age, that related to 'aging' itself and in women, that due to gonadal deficiency. Bone loss due to gonadal deficiency comprises transient and steady-state losses.

PATTERNS OF LOSS

Age loss begins

It is not quite certain when bone loss due to aging begins, due to the lack of prospective studies, but it is believed by some, largely on the basis of cross-sectional studies, to start in both sexes in the 30s. This age-related loss of bone has been compared to the loss of other functions with age, for example, that of muscle mass. Indeed, when bone mineral density of the distal forearm is adjusted for lean body mass, the age-related decreases in bone mineral disappear (Fig. 2.12).

Decline in physical activity

This suggests that the major component of age-related bone loss could relate to the decline in physical activity and is an appropriate functional decrease in skeletal mass. The rate of bone loss in healthy men is low, probably in the order of 3–5% per decade, which partly explains the rather low incidence of osteoporotic fractures in men.

In women the process is more complicated. Bone loss before the menopause is small and probably parallel to that of men. The view

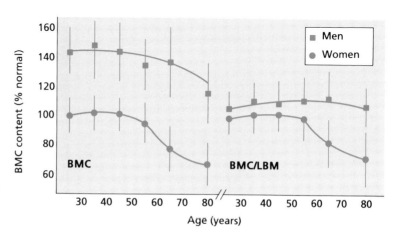

Fig. 2.12 Forearm bone mineral content (BMC; percentage of normal ±1 SD) as a function of age in men and women. The difference between sexes disappears when mass is adjusted for lean body mass (LBM) except after the age of 50 years. (From Thomsen et al., 1986.)

that substantial loss of bone occurs in women well before the age of the menopause is derived from population studies or the use of inadequate methodology. Other prospective studies do not substantiate this view and suggest that if losses in women occur before the menopause, they are very small (Recker *et al.*, 1992).

Menopause

A great deal of evidence indicates the causal relationship between the menopause and accelerated loss of bone. After oophorectomy rapid losses of bone occur which arc prevented by treatment with oestrogens (see Chapter 6). Around the menopause, bone loss accelerates and averages 2% per year over the next 5–10 years and thereafter declines in rate. An early menopause is associated with a low bone mass. The bone mass of women in their 50s who had a premature menopause 20 years earlier is significantly less than that of age-matched menstruating women (Richelson *et al.*, 1984). Moreover, a

Premature menopause

premature menopause is associated with an increase in the risk of hip fracture.

The loss of bone after the menopause is not uniform. Average

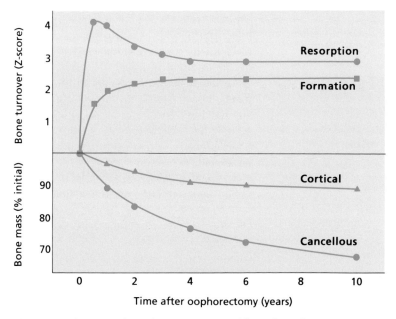

Fig. 2.13 Schema to show the components of bone loss after oophorectomy. The top panel shows biochemical changes in bone resorption (hydroxyproline and tartrate-resistant acid phosphatase) and formation (bone-derived alkaline phosphatase) measured after surgery. The area between these represents the skeletal deficit induced by the increase in turnover. The units are all in SD units (Z-score). The lower panel shows bone loss at a cortical site (the metacarpal) and at the lumbar spine. Note the accelerated losses after surgery which are greater at the spine than in cortical bone related to the increase in activation frequency. After 4 years a new steady state is reached where the rate of loss is constant representing losses due to imbalances at remodelling sites. (Based on Stepan *et al.*, 1987.)

losses based on cross-sectional studies suggest that these are approximately 10% per decade, but level off after the age of 75 years to approach 3% per decade. The short duration of prospective studies and the cross-sectional nature of other studies characterizing bone loss involves many assumptions which in general result in an underestimate of the rate of bone loss, so that characterization of the pattern of loss will require longer term prospective data. The major component of the early bone loss occurring immediately at the time of the menopause is related to an increase in the rate of bone remodelling and the consequences which derive therefrom (see Chapter 1). Superimposed on age-related losses are the additional losses incurred by the imbalance between resorption and formation (Fig. 2.13), so that bone loss continues even when the new steady state has been achieved, proportional to the increase in activation frequency of bone.

On this basis it would be expected that activators of bone turnover would accelerate bone loss and conversely that factors which decrease the activation of turnover would attenuate bone loss. This may explain why rates of loss are higher in women with coexisting hyperparathyroidism and thyrotoxicosis. It also provides a plausible mechanism for accelerated losses due to low calcium diets and during immobilization.

Although bone loss occurs at all sites including the head, arms, hands, chest, spine, pelvis and legs (Gotfredsen *et al.*, 1990), the amount is not uniform. During the early postmenopausal years the amount of bone lost from the peripheral skeletal (largely cortical bone) differs from that lost from the axial skeleton (mainly cancellous bone) and, for example, the rate of bone loss is more rapid at the spine than at the forearm (Fig. 2.14).

The rate of bone loss in the first 10 postmenopausal years also varies widely. It ranges from less than 1% to more than 5% per year. On this basis, postmenopausal women have been stratified into 'normal' and 'fast bone losers' who may be particularly vulnerable to osteoporotic fractures in later life (Hansen *et al.*, 1991). As is the

Early bone loss

Sites of bone loss

Spine

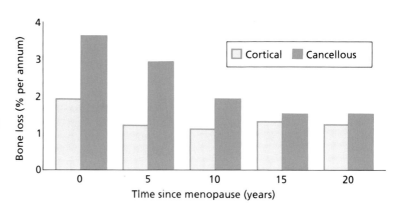

Fig. 2.14 Average rates of bone loss in postmenopausal women assessed at cortical sites (midradius, metacarpal) or predominantly cancellous sites (spine, distal radius) calculated from a literature survey. (Data from C. Slemenda & C. Johnston, personal communication.)

case for peak bone mass, there is, however, no firm evidence to suggest that the distribution of bone loss is truly bimodal.

The factors that determine the rate of bone loss after the menopause are incompletely understood because of the paucity of prospective studies examining losses through the natural menopause or shortly thereafter. There are, however, many factors which have been proposed.

AGE

The age-related loss of bone that occurs in men has been plausibly, but not yet causally, related to the decreasing amount of physical activity with advancing age. This may also explain any modest degree of bone loss that occurs in women before the menopause. On the other hand, the menopause is not a sudden event but a progressive loss of ovarian function that occurs for some years before the cessation of menstrual periods. Thus, in the absence of large prospective studies it is difficult to determine the relative importance of age-related loss compared to other reasons for bone loss.

OESTROGENIC STATUS

Oestrogen deficiency

The degree of oestrogen deficiency is an important factor determining the rate of bone loss, and castrated women lose bone more rapidly than women undergoing a natural menopause. This is probably because bone remodelling is activated more rapidly, but the ultimate effect on bone density when a new steady state is achieved is likely to be small, even though it will have occurred more rapidly. Evidence for this view comes from studies comparing bone mass in women with a natural and premature surgical menopause after 3–20 years. Bone mass is similar in both groups (Richelson *et al.*, 1984).

Oestrogenic status after the menopause (residual ovarian or non-ovarian sources of oestrogen) has an effect on the rate of bone loss. Rates of loss, at least at the appendicular skeleton, correlate with residual oestrogen status in postmenopausal or in oophorectomized women. Population studies have shown variously lower serum values of oestrone, dehydroepiandrostenedione and androstenedione in osteoporosis or in fracture patients than in controls. Others have found no clear relationship between gonadal hormone levels and the rate of bone loss in women after a natural menopause.

Postmenopausal symptoms

There is also a higher frequency of postmenopausal symptoms in patients with vertebral osteoporosis than in controls, and rates of bone loss are greater in those patients with more severe symptoms.

EXERCISE

Prolonged immobilization in the elderly induces bone loss in much the same way as in younger individuals. However, since the balance between formation and resorption is already disturbed in postmeno-pausal women and, since immobilization increases bone turnover, skeletal losses can be considerably accelerated. Some prospective studies have shown that exercise may decrease the rate of bone loss in postmenopausal women (see Chapter 6) but there is little evidence that normal variations in daily physical activity are responsible for variations in rates of bone loss.

NUTRITIONAL FACTORS
As in the case of peak bone mass a variety of nutritional factors have been considered to be important in determining the rate of bone loss. These include high protein, sodium or phosphate diets and a high consumption of caffeine, alcohol and cigarettes (discussed in Chapter 4).

GENETIC FACTORS
There is little evidence that rates of bone loss differ between races (Garn *et al.*, 1969; Matkovic *et al.*, 1979). A recent study has found some differences in postmenopausal rates of bone loss in Norway and Holland. Rates of loss after the menopause appear to be comparable among Japanese, white and black people. Twin and family studies have generally shown that similarities in bone mass become less marked with time, suggesting that the major genetic component is in the determination of peak bone mass rather than rates of bone loss.

Peak bone mass

OBESITY
Obesity is often cited as a protective factor for osteoporosis. The evidence for this is not good, but there is stronger evidence that excessive leanness is a risk factor. The distinction is important since obesity is a risk factor for many other diseases and inappropriate dietary advice may do much harm.

Leanness

Many studies have shown a relationship between body weight and bone mass on hip fracture risk. Those with the higher body weight or higher body mass index (weight/height^2) have the lower risk of fracture. The relationship is, however, not linear, and the increase in risk is confined to the excessively thin. Thinness might affect rates of bone loss because plasma oestrone and oestradiol are proportional to body weight in postmenopausal women, possibly related to the efficacy of conversion of androstenedione to oestrone by adipose tissue (see Chapter 3). However, individuals who weigh more have higher repetitive skeletal loads and the rate of bone loss might be lower for this reason. Thus, the relative contribution of postmeno-pausal body weight, oestrogenic status, body weight and exercise with bone loss is not known.

Determinants of skeletal strength

Bone mass decreases with age at most skeletal sites. The strength of the femoral neck also decreases with age and is lower in women than in men. There is a high correlation between bone mass and bone strength tested *in vitro* (see Chapter 5), and a continuous increase in risk of fracture as bone mass declines.

> Despite this, when individuals with fracture are compared to those of similar age without fracture, there remains overlap in bone mass measurements. This indicates that factors other than low bone mass are important. Such factors may be entirely extraskeletal, such as trauma which occurs in the population, but other skeletal factors may contribute (Table 2B).

Previous fracture

The importance of skeletal abnormalities other than bone mass to overall risk is difficult to assess. The presence of several vertebral fractures considerably increases the risk of subsequent fractures above the risk associated with bone mass alone (see Chapter 1). This finding may be related to changes in mechanical loading of the spine after fractures occur, but could also be related to other intrinsic changes within the bone.

Hip axis length

The geometry of bone is also an important factor. For example, the risk of hip fracture increases with the length of the femoral neck (Faulkner *et al.*, 1993). The effect is independent of bone density and may explain some of the density-independent differences in risk between countries.

Falls

Density-independent components of fracture risk such as falls are clearly important for hip fracture and Colles' fracture but have also been shown for other fractures. For any given bone density, the risk of any of these fractures is greater in the elderly (Hui *et al.*, 1988). The increased frequency of falling, the type of fall which occurs among the elderly, and the loss of protective soft tissue covering may all account for the larger contribution of 'age' and lesser contribution of bone mass which is seen in later life (Hui *et al.*, 1988).

Table 2B Pathogenesis of osteoporotic fracture

Skeletal
Bone mass at maturity
Bone loss
Spatial organization of bone
Turnover of bone
Quality of bone: plasticity, fatigue damage
Shape of bone

Extraskeletal
Falls: frequency, type and severity
Response to trauma – neuromuscular coordination
Soft tissue cushion

Considerable potential energy is generated by falls even from a standing height, and the frequency of falls increases with age. Between the ages of 60 and 64 years the frequency of falls increases from 20% of postmenopausal women to 33% of 80–84 year olds (Cummings & Nevitt, 1989). The frequency of falls is greater in elderly women than in men. The increasing frequency of falls is not sufficient to explain the increasing incidence of fractures with age because only 5–6% of falls give rise to fractures in the elderly. This is due in part to the nature of the fall. For example, the risk of hip fracture is 13 times greater when the point of impact is directly over the hip than elsewhere (Hayes et al., 1991). In addition, the likelihood of fracture is influenced by the thickness of soft tissues over bone which dissipate the force of the fall on impact.

DETERMINANTS OF FRACTURE RISK

In many instances, it is difficult to determine whether a risk factor for fracture arises because of an effect on peak skeletal mass or bone loss. Several observations suggest that environmental factors may be very important in determining the overall risk.

The prevalence of osteoporotic fractures has increased over the past 20 years in all countries where this has been studied, in part due to the increased longevity of the population. Over and above this, the age- and sex-specific incidence of several types of fracture also appears to be increasing in many countries (see Chapter 1). Studies which have shown that age-specific rates have risen in women also show that they have done so in men (see Chapter 1). The marked increase in rates is clearly not explicable on the basis of the menarche or menopause alone. Indeed if anything, the duration of fertile life has increased over this time. In addition, it cannot explain the increase in rates among men. This clearly indicates the importance of factors other than gonadal status in determining changes in hip and other fracture rates within different countries.

Against this background, the incidence of fractures appears to vary markedly from country to country. The most accurate data are available for hip fracture, and rates vary 10-fold throughout the world. As in the case of the secular trend, regional differences in risk affect both men and women. Thus, despite marked sex differences in incidence within centres, age-standardized incidence rates differ more between centres than between sexes (Johnell et al., 1992). Thus, those communities with the higher rates in women are generally those with the higher rates in men. This again suggests that factors other than gonadal status contribute to risk.

A number of factors have been proposed as important determinants of cross-national and international differences. The identification of significant ecological correlates with fracture rates should not be used to argue causality, but nevertheless provide useful information. For example, a late mean menopausal age within a community is

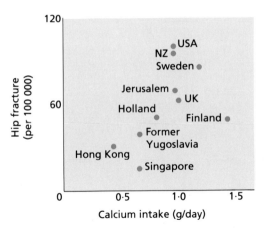

Fig. 2.15 Dietary intake of calcium and the incidence of hip fracture in different countries. (From Kanis & Passmore, 1989.)

associated with a high incidence of hip fracture, though conventional wisdom would indicate that the converse is true in individuals (see Chapter 6). What is clear, however, is that differences in the average age of menopause between communities cannot explain the differences in fracture risk. This apparent paradox between case-control and ecological studies is shared by other putative risk factors such as calcium nutrition. Whereas high doses of calcium delay the rate of bone loss in postmenopausal women and may decrease the risk of fracture (see Chapter 7), there is in ecological terms a direct relationship between calcium intake and hip fracture risk worldwide (Fig. 2.15; Kanis & Passmore, 1989).

Age of menopause

For these reasons, differences in nutritional factors and gonadal status cannot explain the very marked differences in fracture rates around the world. In contrast, both ecological and case-control studies suggest that physical activity is a risk factor within and between communities. As previously mentioned, the average energy expenditure has decreased in many countries, and may have resulted in a progressive decrease of bone capital in successive generations. This is a hypothesis, but if true, it has marked implications for public health, since it implies that the risk of osteoporotic fracture could be decreased markedly by increasing the habitual exposure to physical exercise throughout the community.

Decreased energy expenditure

References

Aaron JE, Francis RM, Peacock M *et al.* (1989) Contrasting microanatomy of idiopathic and corticosteroid-induced osteoporosis. *Clin Orthop*; **243**: 294–305.

Anderson JJB, Tylavsky FA (1984) Diet and osteopenia in elderly Caucasian women. In Christiansen C, Arnaud CD, Nordin BEC, Parfitt AM, Peck WA, Riggs BL (eds). *Osteoporosis*, pp. 299–303. Glostrap Hospital, Copenhagen.

Bonjour J-P, Thientz G, Buchs B, Slosman D, Rizzoli R (1991) Critical years and stages of puberty for spinal and femoral bone mass accumulation during adolescence. *J Clin Endocrinol Metab*; **73**: 555–563.

Boyce WJ, Vessey MP (1985) Rising incidence of fracture of the proximal femur. *Lancet*; **i**: 150–151.

Cummings SR, Nevitt MC (1989) Epidemiology of hip fractures and falls. In Kleerekoper M, Krane SM (eds). *Clinical Disorders of Bone and Mineral Metabolism*, pp. 231–236. Mary Ann Liebert Inc, Publishers, New York.

Drinkwater BL, Chesnut CH (1991) Bone density changes during pregnancy and lactation in active women: a longitudinal study. *Bone Miner*; **14**: 153–160.

Drinkwater BL, Nilson K, Chesnut CH, Bremner WJ, Shainholtz S, Southworth M (1984) Bone mineral content of amenorrheic and eumenorrheic athletes. *N Engl J Med*; **311**: 277–281.

Eriksen EF (1986) Normal and pathological remodelling of human trabecular bone: three-dimensional reconstruction of the remodelling sequence in normals and in metabolic bone disease. *Endocrine Rev*; **7**: 379–408.

Faulkner KG, Cummings SR, Black D, Palermo L, Gluer CC, Genant HK (1993) Simple measurement of femoral geometry predicts hip fracture: the study of osteoporotic fractures. *J Bone Min Res*; **8**: 1211–1217.

Frisch RE, von Gotz-Welbergen A, McArthur JW *et al.* (1981) Delayed menarche and amenorrhea of college athletes in relation to age of onset of training. *JAMA*; **246**: 1559–1563.

Frost HM (1992) The role of changes in mechanical usage set points in the pathogenesis of osteoporosis. *J Bone Miner Res*; **7**: 253–261.

Gardsell PH, Johnell O, Nilsson BE, Serbo I (1991) Bone mass in an urban and a rural population: a comparative, population-based study in southern Sweden. *J Bone Miner Res*; **6**: 67–75.

Garn SM (1970) *The Earlier Gain and Later Loss of Cortical Bone*, pp. 38–55. Charles C Thomas, Springfield.

Garn SM, Rothman CG, Wagner B, Davila GH, Ascoli W (1969) Population similarities in the onset and rate of adult endosteal bone loss. *Clin Orthop*; **65**: 51–60.

Gotfredsen A, Hassager C, Christiansen C (1990) Total and regional bone mass in healthy and osteoporotic women. In Yasumura S, Harrison JE, McNeill KG, Woodhead AD, Dilmanian FA (eds). *Advances in in vivo Body Composition Studies*, pp. 101–106. Plenum Press, New York.

Hansen M, Overgaard K, Riis B, Christiansen C (1991) Role of peak bone mass and bone loss in postmenopausal osteoporosis: 12 year study. *BMJ*; **303**: 961–964.

Hayes WC, Piazza SJ, Zysset PK (1991) Biomechanics of fracture risk prediction of the hip and spine by quantitative computed tomography. *Radiol Clin North Am*; **29(1)**: 1–18.

Hayslip CC, Klein TA, Wray HL, Duncan WL (1989) The effects of lactation on bone mineral content in healthy postpartum women. *Obstet Gynecol*; **73**: 588–592.

Heaney RP, Recker RR, Saville PD (1977) Menopausal changes in calcium balance performance. *J Lab Clin Med*; **92**: 953–963.

Hui SL, Slemenda CS, Johnston CC (1988) Age and bone mass as predictors of fracture in a prospective study. *J Clin Invest*; **81**: 1804–1809.

Johnell O, Gullberg B, Allender E, Kanis JA and the MEDOS study group (1992) The apparent incidence of hip fracture in Europe. *Osteoporosis Int*; **2**: 298–302.

Johnston CC, Norton J, Khairi MRA *et al.* (1985) Heterogeneity of fracture syndromes in postmenopausal women. *J Clin Endocr Metab*; **61**: 551–556.

Johnston CC, Miller JZ, Slemenda CW *et al.* (1992) Calcium supplementation and increases in bone mineral density in children. *N Engl J Med*; **327**: 82–87.

Kanis JA (1991a) *Pathophysiology and Treatment of Paget's Disease of Bone*. Martin Dunitz, London.

Kanis JA (1991b) Calcium requirements for optimal skeletal health in women. *Calcif Tissue Int*; **49** (suppl.): 33–41.

Kanis JA, Passmore R (1989) Calcium supplementation of the diet. *BMJ*; **298**: 137–140, 205–208, 673–674.

Lips P, Netelenbos JC, Jongen MJM *et al.* (1982) Histomorphometric profile and vitamin D status in patients with femoral neck fracture. *Metab Bone Dis Rel Res*; **4**: 85–93.

Matkovic V (1991) Calcium metabolism and calcium requirements during skeletal modelling and consolidation. *Am J Clin Nutr*; **54**: 245–260.

Matkovic V, Kostial K, Simonovic I, Buzina R, Brodarec A, Nordin BEC (1979) Bone status and fracture rates in two regions of Yugoslavia. *Am J Clin Nutr*; **32**: 540–549.

Melton LJ (1990) Fluoride in the prevention of osteoporosis and fractures. *J Bone Miner Res*; **5** (suppl. 1): S163–S167.

Melton LJ (1991) Differing patterns of osteoporosis across the world. In Chesnut CH III (ed.). *New Dimensions in Osteoporosis in the 1990s*, pp. 13–18. Excerpta Medica Asia, Hong Kong.

Melton LJ (1993) Hip fractures: a worldwide problem today and tomorrow. *Bone*; **14** (suppl.): 1–8.

Meunier PJ, Sellami S, Briancon D *et al.* (1981) Histological heterogeneity of apparently idiopathic osteoporosis. In De Luca HF, Frost HM, Jee WSS, Johnston CC, Parfitt AM (eds). *Osteoporosis. Recent Advances in Pathogenesis and Treatment*, pp. 293–301. University Park Press, Baltimore.

Moller M, Horsman A, Harvald B, Hauge M, Henningsen K, Nordin BEC (1978) Metacarpal morphometry in monozygotic and dizygotic elderly twins. *Calcif Tissue Int*; **25**: 197–201.

Mosekilde L, Mosekilde L (1990) Sex differences in age-related changes in vertebral body size, density and biomechanical competence in normal individuals. *Bone*; **11**: 67–73.

Nomura A, Wasnich RD, Heilbrun LK, Ross PD, Davis JW (1989) Comparison of bone mineral content between Japan-born and US-born Japanese subjects in Hawaii. *Bone Miner*; **6**: 213–223.

Nordin BEC, Heaney RP (1990) Calcium supplementation of the diet: justified by the present evidence. *BMJ*; **300**: 1056–1059.

Parfitt AM (1983) The physiological and clinical significance of bone histo-morphometric data. In Recker R (ed.). *Bone Histomorphometry, Techniques and Interpretation*, pp. 143–223. CRC Press, Boca Raton.

Parfitt AM (1987) Trabecular bone architecture in the pathogenesis and prevention of fracture. *Am J Med*; **82** (IB): 68–72.

Parfitt AM, Mathews C, Rao D *et al.* (1981) Impaired osteoblast function in metabolic bone disease. In DeLuca HF, Frost HM, Jee WSS, Johnston CC, Parfitt AM (eds). *Osteoporosis: Recent Advances in Pathogenesis and Treatment*, pp. 321–330. University Park Press, Baltimore.

Parfitt AM, Mathews CHE, Villanueva AR *et al.* (1983) Relationships between surface volume and thickness of iliac trabecular bone in ageing and osteoporosis. *J Clin Invest*; **72**: 1396–1409.

Recker RR, Kimmel DB, Parfitt AM, Davies M, Keshawarz N, Hinders S (1988) Static and tetracycline based bone histomorphometric data from 34 normal postmenopausal females. *J Bone Miner Res*; **3**: 133–144.

Recker RR, Davies M, Hinders M *et al.* (1992) Bone gain in young adults. *J Am Med Assoc*; **268**: 2403–2408.

Richelson LS, Wahner HW, Melton LJ, Riggs BL (1984) Relative contributions of aging and estrogen deficiency to postmenopausal bone loss. *N Engl J Med*; **311**: 1273–1275.

Rubin CT, Lanyon LE (1985) Regulation of bone mass by mechanical strain magnitude. *Calcif Tissue Int*; **37**: 411−417.

Sowers MF, Corton G, Shapiro B *et al.* (1993) Changes in bone density with lactation. *JAMA*; **269**: 3130−3135.

Stepan JJ, Pospichal J, Presl J *et al.* (1987) Bone loss and biochemical indices of bone remodelling in surgically induced postmenopausal women. *Bone*; **8**: 279−284.

Thomsen K, Gotfredsen A, Christiansen G (1986) Is postmenopausal bone loss an age related phenomenon? *Calcif Tissue Int*; **39**: 123−127.

Todd RC, Freeman MAR, Price CJ (1972) Isolated trabecular fatigue fractures in the femoral neck. *J Bone Joint Surg*; **54B**: 723−728.

Trusswell AS, Irwin T, Beaton GH *et al.* (1983) Recommended dietary intake around the world. *Nutrition Abstracts and Review*; **53**: 939−1015.

Vernon-Roberts B, Pirie CJ (1973) Healing trabecular microfractures in the bodies of lumbar vertebrae. *Ann Rheumatic Dis*; **32**: 406−412.

Vesterby A, Mosekilde L, Gundersen HJG *et al.* (1991) Biologically meaningful determinants of the in vitro strength of lumbar vertebrae. *Bone*; **12**: 219−224.

Whyte MP, Bergfeld MA, Murphy WA *et al.* (1982) Postmenopausal osteoporosis: a heterogeneous disorder as assessed by histomorphometric analysis of iliac crest bone from untreated patients. *Am J Med*; **72**: 193−202.

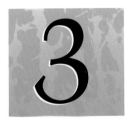

The endocrinology and biochemistry of osteoporosis

The disturbances in calcium homeostasis in most forms of osteoporosis are relatively subtle – as are the disturbances in skeletal metabolism. Notwithstanding, many endocrine abnormalities have been described in osteoporosis and it is often considered as an endocrine disorder. The most obvious of these is the gonadal insufficiency of postmenopausal osteoporosis, but even in this disorder other abnormalities reported include disturbances in the secretion, synthesis or action of parathyroid hormone (PTH), calcitonin, vitamin D, insulin-like growth factors and other hormones. They are often considered to be causes of osteoporosis or at least to contribute to skeletal losses, but the interpretation of the finding of endocrine abnormalities is complex for several reasons.

The first relates to the subtlety of the differences described, so that it is difficult to determine whether they arise from the inadequacy of the control populations studied. Secondly, many changes in hormonal status occur with aging. It is, therefore, important but not always possible to distinguish changes which arise because of age from those of osteoporosis. Finally, the associations are not necessarily causal. For example, some of the changes described in plasma vitamin D metabolism in the postmenopausal years may be consequences rather than the causes of osteoporosis. In addition, several of the abnormalities described are observed after acute dynamic tests and their relevance to the long-term steady-state situation is uncertain. This chapter describes the changes in calcium metabolism reported in osteoporosis against the background of the regulation of calcium homeostasis in health.

Plasma calcium

Fifty percent of the extraskeletal calcium is found in the extracellular fluid (ECF). Changes in the concentration of plasma ionized calcium are usually accompanied by changes in the total amount of calcium in the extracellular fluid since there is a passive distribution of ionized calcium throughout the ECF compartment. Within the plasma compartment, however, approximately 50% of calcium is

bound to proteins, mainly albumin, and the binding is pH dependent
(Table 3.1; Marshall, 1976). In the absence of severe acidosis or
alkalosis, the major factors influencing the amount of calcium bound
is the quantity of albumin present, since the proportion of calcium is
fairly constant. Ionized calcium is ideally measured but is tedious to
perform and requires rapid and anaerobic handling of the samples.
For this reason formulae are used for predicting the ionized calcium
from the total plasma calcium or 'correcting' the total plasma calcium
to a normal protein value. A simple correction factor for plasma
calcium which is widely used is to subtract from (or add to) total
plasma calcium 0.02 mmol/l (0.08 mg/dl) for every gram per litre
that the plasma albumin exceeds (or is less than) 40 g/l, provided
that the sample is drawn without venous stasis.

Although rates of bone formation and resorption are obviously
disrupted in osteoporosis, there are remarkably few changes in plasma
calcium and phosphate metabolism in uncomplicated osteoporosis.
There is a small increase in serum calcium in the immediate postmenopausal state, which appears to be partly due to a change in
protein binding. However, the changes in plasma calcium are small,
and plasma concentrations of calcium (and of phosphate) typically lie
within the laboratory reference range (Table 3.2). If plasma calcium
is abnormal in the presence of osteoporosis this indicates either an

Table 3.1 Distribution of plasma calcium

Ultrafilterable calcium (53%)	
Ionized calcium	47
Complexed calcium (6%)	
Phosphate	1.5
Citrate	1.5
HCO_3 etc.	3
Protein bound calcium (47%)	
Albumin	37
Globulin	10
Total plasma calcium (2.12–2.60 mmol/l)	100%

Table 3.2 Serum calcium fractions (mean ± SD) in women aged 40–50 years
according to menopausal status. (From Sokoll *et al.*, 1988)

	Premenopausal	Postmenopausal
Total serum calcium (mmol/l)	2.27 ± 0.05	2.35 ± 0.05*
Ionized calcium (mmol/l)	1.26 ± 0.02	1.27 ± 0.04
Albumin (g/l)	47 ± 4	45 ± 4

* Significantly different from premenopausal women.

57 / Endocrinology and biochemistry

additional disorder or the presence of a disorder giving rise to a secondary cause of osteoporosis (see Chapter 4).

Calcium transport to and from the ECF

With the exception of the pregnant or lactating female, the major fluxes of calcium to and from the ECF occur across the intestinal mucosa, bone and kidney (Fig. 3.1).

INTESTINE
Calcium normally enters the body only by its intestinal absorption. The true absorption of calcium is greater than the net absorption because some calcium is returned to the gut lumen in biliary, pancreatic and intestinal secretions. Thus, from an average daily dietary

Dietary intake

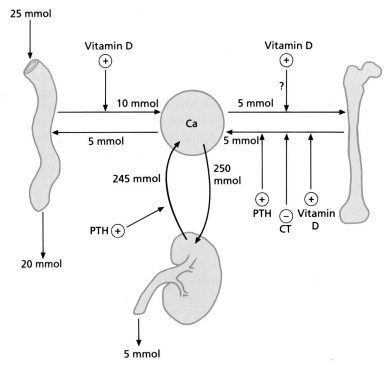

Fig. 3.1 Major fluxes of calcium (mmol/day) in a healthy adult. Exchange of calcium in the extracellular fluid occurs with bone, gut and kidney. The net balance for calcium equals the net absorption minus the losses of calcium in faeces and urine, which in a healthy adult is zero. The major fluxes of calcium are regulated by the regulating hormones. Parathyroid hormone (PTH) increases renal tubular reabsorption of calcium and bone resorption. Calcitonin (CT) inhibits bone resorption and vitamin D augments intestinal absorption for calcium. The precise role of vitamin D in augmenting bone resorption and mineralization *in vivo* is not clear.

intake of 25 mmol (1 g), approximately 10 mmol are absorbed. This is offset by intestinal secretions amounting to approximately 5 mmol (0.2 g) daily, leaving a net transport into the ECF pool of 5 mmol.

> The availability of calcium for absorption depends upon many dietary factors including the presence of phosphate, oxalates, fats and phytates which bind calcium and render it less available for absorption. Calcium in the form of milk or dairy products is generally freely bioavailable, whereas that contained in some green vegetables is less available.

Active transport sites

Absorption occurs throughout the length of the small intestine and depends both on active transport and diffusion processes. The major sites for active transport are in the duodenum and upper part of the jejunum and depend on vitamin D. However, because the duodenum is relatively short compared with the rest of the gastrointestinal tract, more calcium is probably absorbed at sites distal to the duodenum than within the duodenum itself, at least with normal dietary intakes.

Tests for calcium absorption

A variety of tests are available to study calcium absorption (Charles, 1989). Calcium balance provides an index of net calcium transport. Faecal and urinary excretion are measured over a period of several days and then compared with measurement of dietary intake. Accurate assessment of unidirectional fluxes of calcium across the gut is dependent upon the use of tracer techniques. A standard method is to compare the plasma appearance and disappearance of an orally administered calcium isotope with the disappearance of an intravenously given calcium isotope.

A 24-hour urine collection for calcium or phosphate provides an indirect index of intestinal absorption, provided it is assumed or known that the net flux of these ions across bone and other tissues is zero. The expression of excretion as a ratio to creatinine helps to adjust for differences in body weight and for incomplete urine collections.

Disorders of vitamin D metabolism

Increased intestinal absorption of calcium is found in several disease states associated with osteoporosis, such as hyperparathyroidism, sarcoidosis and idiopathic hypercalciuria, and is attributable to increased production of calcitriol. Conversely, malabsorption of calcium may be associated with low levels of calcitriol, for example in hypoparathyroidism, vitamin D deficiency states and chronic renal failure. Malabsorption of calcium also occurs in disorders in which the target tissue for calcitriol is defective. A good example of this is in untreated coeliac disease, where the flat intestinal mucosa lacks the villi and enterocytes through which calcium is normally absorbed.

> Changes in the absorption of calcium and in the metabolism of vitamin D occur with age, and this has led to the view that

osteoporosis may be due in part to impaired metabolism or action of vitamin D.

BONE

In the mature adult who is neither gaining nor losing calcium, bone and soft tissues contribute neither a net gain nor a net loss of calcium from the ECF. Thus, the amount of bone resorbed accounts for approximately 5 mmol of calcium daily, and exactly matches the amount of bone formed.

Studies with radioisotopes (calcium and strontium isotopes) have shown that in normal human adults there is a large exchangeable pool of calcium between bone and the ECF. This exchangeable pool of calcium is important in plasma calcium homeostasis (Staub *et al.*, 1989), but should be distinguished from the movements of calcium that occur in bone as a result of mineralization and bone resorption, which account for only a fraction of the total calcium exchange.

Provided that serum calcium is stable, the total excretion of calcium reflects the net input of calcium to the ECF, largely from gut and skeletal sources. If patients are in the fasting state (usually overnight) and urine collected thereafter in the postabsorptive state, the urinary excretion more closely reflects net efflux of calcium from bone. A 2-hour urine collection is commonly used, but the timing is not critical if the urinary excretion is expressed as the calcium/creatinine ratio. Fasting urinary excretion of calcium is high in osteoporosis and decreases with effective treatment. More specific indices of bone turnover are reviewed in Chapter 5.

KIDNEY

The kidney is a major site for calcium excretion from the body. A large amount of calcium is filtered (see Fig. 3.1) and most of this is reabsorbed so that only 1–3% is excreted into the urine. These large fluxes through the kidney to and from the ECF compartment mean that small changes in renal tubular reabsorption may have profound effects on the ECF concentration of calcium. Since reabsorption is under hormonal control, principally by PTH, this has led to the view that the kidney is a major organ in the regulation of plasma calcium.

In osteoporosis an increase in bone resorption increases serum calcium which in turn suppresses the secretion of PTH and decreases renal tubular reabsorption of calcium. The greater the rate of bone resorption the greater the effect. This decrease in tubular reabsorption offsets the effect of the hypercalcaemic challenge and is an important sparing mechanism. Thus, the presence of hypercalcaemia in osteoporosis usually denotes either massive osteolysis or the secretion of hormones such as PTH or PTH-related peptide (PTHrP), which themselves increase renal tubular reabsorption of calcium.

Bone resorption

Fasting state

Renal tubular reabsorption

Calcium excretion is influenced by other factors, notably sodium excretion, ECF volume, and the administration of diuretics (Kleeman *et al.*, 1964). Infusion of sodium chloride increases the excretion of calcium, an effect which probably contributes to its value in the acute treatment of hypercalcaemia. A high sodium diet has for this reason been suggested as a cause for nephrolithiasis and osteoporosis (see Chapter 4).

Calcium balance is a function of the integrated fluxes across bone, gut and kidney. These fluxes are continually changing and are affected by a variety of factors including several hormones. These hormones can be subdivided into 'controlling' and 'influencing' hormones. The

controlling hormones are the major regulating hormones, PTH, calcitonin and the vitamin D metabolites, the secretion of each of which is altered in response to changes in plasma ionized calcium

concentrations. The influencing hormones are those other hormones such as thyroid hormones, growth hormones and adrenal and gonadal steroids which have important effects on calcium metabolism but whose secretion is determined primarily by factors other than changes in plasma calcium.

PTH

In the circulation, PTH consists of several polypeptide fragments which are degraded in the liver and kidney. The major stimulus to the secretion of PTH is a fall in the ionized fraction of plasma calcium. The biological actions of PTH at a variety of target organs serve to increase the plasma calcium concentration, which in turn suppresses the secretion of PTH, so that there exists an efficient negative-feedback hormonal loop (Fitzpatrick *et al.*, 1992).

The target organ actions of PTH include effects on bone, kidney and indirectly on gut. PTH acts on the kidney to increase the tubular reabsorption of calcium and to depress the tubular reabsorption of phosphate (Peacock & Nordin, 1968). This induces a rise in plasma calcium and a fall in plasma phosphate. PTH also stimulates the 1α-hydroxylase enzyme responsible for the production of calcitriol, leading to increased intestinal absorption of calcium and possibly to the release of calcium from bone. Thus, many of the actions of PTH on the kidney appear either directly or indirectly to increase the ECF concentration of calcium.

Mammalian PTH consists of a single peptide chain containing 84 amino acids, but only the first 32–34 amino acids (reading from the N-terminal end) are necessary for biological activity. Cleavage occurs naturally, partly in the liver, to produce a short N-terminal biologically active fragment and a larger inactive C-terminal fragment. This cleavage may be necessary for PTH to act on bone. There are also many less well characterized circulating fragments of PTH. The liver and kidney are important sites of their degradation and fragments normally cleared by the kidney may be increased in chronic renal failure, though the circulating biological activity of PTH may be normal. This causes some problems in the interpretation of radio-immunoassay in patients with renal impairment. Several assays have been developed to detect specific sequences such as the amino-terminal portion of the molecule or intact PTH which partially resolve the problem.

Pulsatile secretion of PTH

Studies using assays to detect the intact hormone have shown that the secretion of PTH is normally pulsatile. Studies in the elderly suggest that this pulsatility is lost or at least blunted. Because PTH may have anabolic effects on some aspects of skeletal metabolism (see Chapter 8), the blunting of pulsatility has been used to argue that this contributes to the process of osteoporosis (Hesch *et al.*, 1989), and that the intermittent use of PTH might therefore reverse the pathogenetic mechanism. It is not clear, however, whether loss of pulsatility contributes to bone loss. Moreover, it is not clear whether the phenomenon is related to aging or other factors rather than specifically to osteoporosis.

Oestrogen

Oestrogen appears to alter the set-point around which calcium stimulates the secretion of PTH. In this regard it is of interest that primary hyperparathyroidism commonly presents in women at the time of the menopause, and indeed can be treated with either oestrogens or progestogens (Selby & Peacock, 1986). This suggests that gonadal steroids alter the set-point for serum calcium homeostasis either by an influence on the parathyroid gland or on the target tissues which determine the set-point. The latter seems more likely since neither oestrogen deficiency nor oestrogens, when given to oestrogen-deficient women, appear to alter the secretion of PTH. In addition, the administration of oestrogens increases urinary excretion of nephrogenous cyclic adenosine monophosphate (cAMP) (Stock *et al.*, 1988) and decreases renal tubular reabsorption of phosphate without altering PTH values, suggesting increased renal sensitivity to PTH.

Renal function

Renal function declines with age, which may affect PTH metabolism. Levels of PTH increase with age (Gallagher *et al.*, 1979). It is possible that intrinsic renal damage to the 1α-hydroxylase impairs production of calcitriol, decreases intestinal absorption of calcium, lowers serum calcium and stimulates the secretion of PTH in much the same way as early in the development of renal bone disease. Additionally, secondary hyperparathyroidism may be induced by vitamin D deficiency. Marked or persistent vitamin D deficiency will eventually result in osteomalacia and contribute independently to skeletal fragility.

Calcitonin

Calcitonin is produced mainly by the C-cells of the thyroid in humans. It is a peptide hormone containing 32 amino acid residues with a disulphide bridge between cysteine residues in positions 1 and 7. The entire sequence is essential for biological activity and the gene structure of the human hormone has been elaborated. There are several differences in the amino acid composition of the calcitonins from different species and these are associated with different potencies.

Circulates in heterogeneous form

Calcitonin circulates in plasma in heterogeneous form, which causes many problems in evaluating its biological function as well as its role in the pathogenesis of osteoporosis, since values measured by radioimmunoassay vary widely, and some qualitative as well as quantitative differences are found between centres. The development of assays which measure monomeric 1–32 calcitonin has not resolved these problems, and there is much conflicting evidence as to how calcitonin secretion responds to various 'physiological' stresses.

Action of calcitonin

Many agents affect the secretion of calcitonin (Azria, 1989). These include calcium, gastrointestinal hormones such as cholecystokinin, enteroglucagon and gastrin, β-adrenergic agents and alcohol. An obvious action of calcitonin is to inhibit bone resorption and thereby lower plasma calcium, so that it is widely believed that calcitonin is a calcium-regulating hormone with a negative-feedback mechanism.

Osteoclasts and calcitonin

Exposure of osteoclasts to calcitonin causes invagination of the brush border, retraction from the bone surface and a decrease in their motility (Chambers & Magnus, 1982). Although the most obvious action of calcitonin in mammals is to inhibit bone resorption, it also has effects at other sites. In the kidney it decreases renal tubular reabsorption of calcium, phosphate, magnesium, potassium, and a variety of other ions, and is a powerful diuretic. It also inhibits the secretion of several gastrointestinal hormones. A further action of calcitonin that may have relevance to its use in symptomatic osteoporosis is its analgesic properties. The mechanism for this effect is controversial, but could be a direct central effect of the drug or mediated by an increase in endogenous opiate secretion.

Despite the many effects of calcitonin, it is difficult to ascribe a physiological role for this hormone. One difficulty is that a deficiency (total thyroidectomy) or excess (medullary carcinoma of the thyroid) of calcitonin is associated with only minor disturbances in skeletal or mineral homeostasis.

Physiological role

Serum values of calcitonin and its response to provocative tests such as calcium infusions have been variously described as normal or low in osteoporosis. Studies of the endogenous secretion rate of calcitonin have shown that this may also be impaired (Reginster *et al.*, 1989). They have also been described as lower in women than in men. An inference deriving from such studies is that in women, calcitonin reserves may be inadequate to protect against skeletal losses irrespective of the initiating events to cause bone loss (e.g., oestrogen deficiency). Low values have been shown to increase after the administration of exogenous oestrogens and may be a direct effect. This has been used to further argue that oestrogen deficiency gives rise to calcitonin deficiency which in turn accelerates the activation frequency of bone. Not all studies, however, show an effect of oestrogens on calcitonin secretion. Other findings including a blunted calcitonin response following provocative tests such as calcium infusion are not invariant.

> Thus, the notion that osteoporosis is due to calcitonin deficiency is far from proven. This conclusion does not infer that calcitonin should not be of value in the management of bone loss (see Chapter 7). However, the doses of calcitonin used in therapeutics are pharmacological.

Vitamin D

Sources of vitamin D

Vitamin D_3 (cholecalciferol) is derived from the diet, and from the skin by ultraviolet irradiation of 7-dehydrocholesterol. Vitamin D_2 (ergocalciferol) is a product originally derived from the ultraviolet irradiation of plant sterols and is used to supplement the diet. In many respects vitamin D_2 and D_3 are comparable in their metabolism and in their actions.

Metabolic conversions

Calcidiol

Before exerting biological effects, vitamin D undergoes a series of further metabolic conversions (Fig. 3.2; Henry & Norman, 1992). The first step involves its conversion in the liver to a 25-hydroxylated derivative (25-OHD; calcidiol). This is the major circulating vitamin D metabolite, and is the metabolite most commonly measured clinically to provide an index of vitamin D nutritional status. In northern latitudes there is a marked seasonal variation in plasma 25-OHD levels with a peak in late summer and a trough in late winter. In winter, plasma levels may commonly approach those associated with vitamin D-deficiency states, suggesting that in northern Europe both sunlight and dietary intake may be of crucial importance in maintaining vitamin D status.

Calcitriol/secalciferol

The second step in the metabolism of vitamin D is its further hydroxylation, mainly in the kidney, to either 1,25-dihydroxy vitamin D_3 (calcitriol) or to $24,25(OH)_2D_3$ (secalciferol). The renal metabolism of calcitriol is closely regulated, and its production is favoured under conditions of deficiency of vitamin D, calcium or phosphate. Production of calcitriol is also augmented by a variety of hormones, including oestradiol, prolactin and growth hormone, but it is not clear if this is a direct effect of the hormones on the kidney or if it is mediated by changes in calcium or phosphate concentration.

> Of the major metabolites of vitamin D, calcitriol has the greatest biological potency in many experimental systems studied

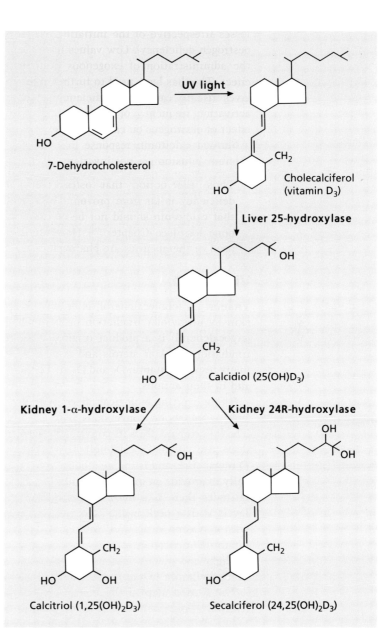

Fig. 3.2 Steps in the conversion of 7-dehydrocholesterol to vitamin D and its metabolites. The site of synthesis of 25-hydroxyvitamin D_3 (calcidiol; 25(OH)D_3) is in the liver. The active form of vitamin D (calcitriol; 1,25(OH)$_2D_3$) is made in the kidney and placenta. Secalciferol (24,25(OH)$_2D_3$) is synthesized in several tissues, but the kidney is probably the major site.

Within the figure:

UV light

7-Dehydrocholesterol

HO

Cholecalciferol (vitamin D_3)

CH_2

HO

Liver 25-hydroxylase

OH

Calcidiol (25(OH)D_3)

CH_2

HO

Kidney 1-α-hydroxylase

Kidney 24R-hydroxylase

OH

OH

CH_2

HO OH

Calcitriol (1,25(OH)$_2D_3$)

OH

OH

CH_2

HO

Secalciferol (24,25(OH)$_2D_3$)

(DeLuca, 1990). Its principal effects are to increase intestinal absorption of calcium and phosphate and to increase the resorption of calcium from bone. Although lack of vitamin D in humans is associated with defective mineralization of cartilage and bone, it is still not known whether vitamin D and its metabolites act directly on bone to promote its mineralization (Kanis *et al.*, 1982).

Despite the presence of calcitriol receptors on osteoblasts, and the production of bone-specific proteins such as osteocalcin in response to vitamin D, it is possible that the effects of vitamin D on bone mineralization are secondary to changes in ECF concentrations of calcium and phosphate. From a teleological viewpoint, the action of calcitriol can be thought of as increasing the availability of calcium and phosphate for mineralization, or as maintaining plasma levels of calcium and phosphate.

Calcitriol can therefore be considered to be the hormonal form of vitamin D, in the sense that its secretion from endocrine tissue (the kidney) is controlled by the calcium and phosphate status of the individual, and that the action of this hormone reverses the stimulus to its secretion.

Mechanisms for calcium malabsorption

Many studies have reported a decrease in the serum concentration of calcitriol in the early postmenopausal period. On this basis it has been suggested that this gives rise to intestinal malabsorption of calcium (Gallagher *et al.*, 1979) which, in view of the increased requirement for calcium after the menopause, accelerates osteoporotic bone loss (Fig. 3.3). Since oestrogens may stimulate the synthesis of calcitriol at least *in vitro*, oestrogen withdrawal is thought to be the signal for decreased production of calcitriol. This is not, however, the only possible mechanism to account for calcium

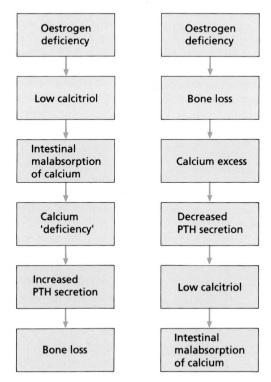

Fig. 3.3 Schema to show the different mechanisms for bone loss and their relationship to calcium absorption. The sequence shown on the left hypothesizes that a decrease in intestinal absorption of calcium augments bone loss whereas that on the right suggests that a decrease in intestinal absorption of calcium is a consequence of bone loss. PTH, parathyroid hormone.

malabsorption. It is equally plausible that oestrogen deficiency directly causes bone loss, which in turn infuses the ECF with calcium, and that this in turn decreases the secretion of PTH and the synthesis of calcitriol. Thus, the intestinal malabsorption is a consequence of the bone loss and not its cause (see Fig. 3.3).

Hyperparathyroidism of aging

With advancing years, lower values for calcitriol and increased secretion of PTH are found (Gallagher *et al.*, 1979). Both changes could well be due to the decline in renal function with age. Others, on the basis of population studies, suggest that hyperparathyroidism is common in the postmenopausal population and that hyperparathyroidism is due to vitamin D deficiency. Several studies have examined the responsivity of the 1α-hydroxylase to PTH and found this to be impaired, but not more so in osteoporotic patients than in others. This suggests that abnormalities in vitamin D metabolism with aging occur, but that they are a generalized phenomenon rather than specific for an osteoporotic population. The various mechanisms whereby secondary hyperparathyroidism might occur and its inter-relationship with vitamin D are shown in Figure 3.4.

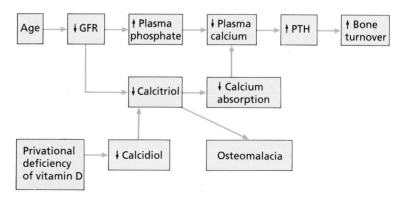

Fig. 3.4 Schema for the pathogenesis of secondary hyperparathyroidism with age. As renal function declines with age, this increases the phosphate load per nephron and induces a fall in serum calcium, in turn stimulating the secretion of parathyroid hormone (PTH). PTH secretion tends to reverse changes in plasma calcium and phosphate (renal action). As renal function declines, plasma calcium and phosphate remain relatively normal but at the expense of an ever increasing secretion of PTH and its skeletal consequences – an increase in activation frequency of bone. Low concentrations of calcitriol arise because of the decline in renal function and impair intestinal absorption of calcium and aggravate hyperparathyroidism. This effect may be augmented in the presence of privational vitamin D deficiency. Long-standing vitamin D deficiency additionally induces osteomalacia. Some investigators have additionally suggested that the response of intestinal tissue to calcitriol is impaired with age or with osteoporosis.

Integrated effects

Calcium homeostasis

In considering calcium homeostasis, it is useful to draw some distinction between the way in which the plasma calcium is set at a particular concentration, and the way in which movements of calcium in and out of ECF are adjusted (Staub *et al.*, 1989). The plasma calcium level is set close to a particular value in different individuals in normal and disease states. The set-point can be defined as the mean serum calcium of an individual and the SD, the efficiency with which the set-point is maintained. This efficiency is not markedly disturbed in osteoporosis. Deviations from the set-point rather than the set-point itself are corrected in part, but not exclusively, by hormone-induced changes in all the fluxes of calcium to and from the ECF compartment.

When the system is disturbed, a steady state no longer exists, and the response which occurs adjusts the system so that a new steady state comes into existence.

Disruption of steady state

An example of a disruption of the steady state in osteoporosis is the increase in bone turnover that occurs after the menopause. This results in an increase in delivery of calcium to the ECF analogous to an infusion of calcium. During the calcium infusion, the plasma calcium concentration will begin to rise. If the rate of calcium infusion is constant, levels of plasma calcium will not rise indefinitely but only until the rate of efflux of calcium from the extracellular pool (to bone, kidney, gut and other tissues) matches the rate of influx. At this point, plasma calcium levels will not rise further, despite continuing the infusion, and a new steady state prevails. In practice, the rise in plasma calcium during a calcium infusion is to some extent buffered by the exchange of calcium in bone, and any increase in serum calcium will result in the suppression of secretion of PTH and a decrease in the renal tubular reabsorption for calcium. This will increase urinary losses of calcium and tend to increase the rate at which a new steady state is achieved. Thus, rises or falls in plasma calcium are partially compensated by increased net movements of calcium into or out of bone.

The response to prolonged perturbations of serum calcium brings in contributions from changes in vitamin D metabolism, and from the intestine and bone. An example is the adaptation that occurs to a change in dietary intake of calcium. If intake is markedly increased, this will tend to cause an increase in plasma calcium which will decrease the secretion of PTH. Apart from its effects on the kidney, a sustained decrease in PTH will lead both to decreased resorption of bone, and to a decrease in synthesis of calcitriol. This in turn will decrease intestinal absorption of calcium and perhaps resorption of calcium from bone. If the increase in dietary calcium continues,

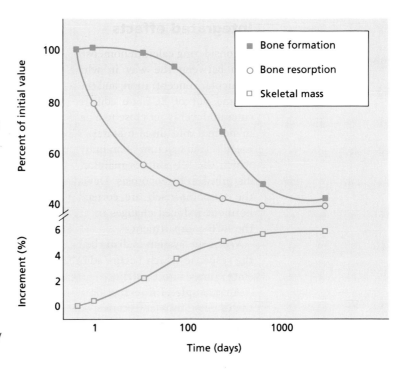

Fig. 3.5 Effect of a prolonged and high dietary intake of calcium on bone resorption and formation, and skeletal mass. Note the earlier decrease in bone resorption followed later by a decrease in formation due to coupling. Bone mass increases during the transient phase until formation rates are decreased to match those of resorption. In the new steady state, bone mass no longer changes but is higher than before the dietary manipulation.

New steady state

these changes will act to restore the plasma calcium towards its previous value, and the bone formation rate will decrease to match the rate of decreased bone resorption by the coupling mechanism. The new steady state will consist of a lower efficiency of intestinal absorption of calcium and a decreased rate of entry and removal of calcium from bone, so that a net balance can be maintained, albeit with a slightly increased skeletal mass (Fig. 3.5).

Gonadal steroids and the endocrinology of the menopause

Characteristic growth abnormalities are associated with deficiencies of either male or female sex hormones. They appear to play a crucial role in epiphyseal closure and in the adolescent growth spurt which precedes this event. They may also influence the amount of calcium present in the skeleton in adult life. In adults the effects of oestrogens are of particular interest because of the loss of bone that occurs in women after the menopause. A great deal of evidence (see Chapters 2, 4 and 6) indicates that postmenopausal bone loss is causally related to the decline in ovarian function that occurs at the time of the menopause.

THE MENOPAUSE

Definition

The menopause is defined as the last physiological menstrual bleed from the endometrium. It is thus a retrospective diagnosis. For practical purposes it is generally acknowledged as the absence of menses for 6–12 months and can be confirmed by persistently increased serum values for follicle-stimulating hormone or luteinizing hormone.

Climacteric

Whereas the menopause describes the cessation of menses, ovarian function declines for several years beforehand and is termed the climacteric. During this period, the production of progesterone by the corpora lutea begins to fall and the interval between cycles lengthens, resulting in less regular bleeds. This 'hypoluteal phase' is followed later by a decrease in ovarian production of oestrogen. Menstrual abnormalities are common in the 10 years before the menopause and may present as heavy bleeding, intermenstrual spotting or painful periods due to failing progesterone production. More often, periods become less frequent and associated with less blood loss. Although fertility decreases markedly during the climacteric, the risk of pregnancy is sufficient that contraception, if practised, should be continued until the diagnosis of the menopause is established.

Age of menopause

Ovarian follicles

The age at menopause is thought to be related to the number of ovarian follicles produced during fetal development, which in turn may be genetically determined (Goecke, 1959). Peak numbers occur before birth and decline throughout life. The rate of attrition of ovarian follicles is high. Of the 5 million or so at birth, several hundred thousand follicles remain at sexual maturity, and ovarian endocrine failure occurs when follicle numbers decrease to less than 1000. The factors that govern the normal attrition of ovarian follicles are not known. The average age of the menopause is at 51 years in the

Average age

Western world, but there are small but significant differences between communities. The age appears to occur later in countries with higher socioeconomic development. These are generally countries with the higher incidence of osteoporotic hip fracture.

> The paradoxical situation arises therefore that a later age of menopause in a community is associated with an increased risk of fracture, but within communities an early menopause increases the risk. The increase in risk associated with a late menopausal age is doubtless confounded by other factors such as socioeconomic status and exercise.

The age of the menopause is not apparently influenced by prolonged periods of amenorrhoea, the number of pregnancies or the use of oral contraceptives. Dogma would have it that the age of the menopause has changed little since antiquity, but this is unlikely to be true. Notwithstanding, the age of the menopause has changed little com-

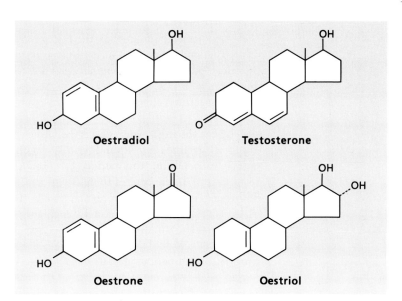

Fig. 3.6 Chemical structure of some gonadal steroids.

pared with the survival of women so that, with time, progressively more of the female population is postmenopausal and progressively more of a woman's life is spent in the postmenopausal state.

Apart from genetic potential and socioeconomic status there are few factors known to affect the age of menopause. Smoking has been suggested to accelerate the age of menopause, but the evidence for this is unconvincing. There are, however, other reasons to consider smoking as a risk factor (see Chapter 4).

Ovarian oestrogen production

Forms of oestrogen

During fertile life the ovaries are the major source of circulating oestrogens. The major forms of oestrogen of significance are oestrone (E_1), oestradiol (E_2), and oestriol (E_3) (Fig. 3.6). Of these oestradiol is the most potent, but circulates at lower concentrations than oestrone. Oestriol is even less potent and is primarily produced by the metabolic conversion of oestradiol and oestrone. High serum concentrations of oestriol are found only during pregnancy. Before the menopause 90% of circulating oestradiol is ovarian in origin. About 10% is produced by the non-ovarian conversion of oestrone, androstenedione and testosterone, mainly in adipose tissue.

The menopause is associated with major changes in the production of oestrogens, androgens and progestogens (Table 3.3 and Fig. 3.7).

Decline in oestradiol production

Since the ovary is the major site of production of oestradiol, the menopause is associated with a marked decrease in its concentration. Plasma levels fall to about 10% of those found before the menopause. Some residual oestradiol is ovarian but most is derived from androgens, and serum levels are similar in oophorectomized women and in those who have undergone a natural menopause. The pro-

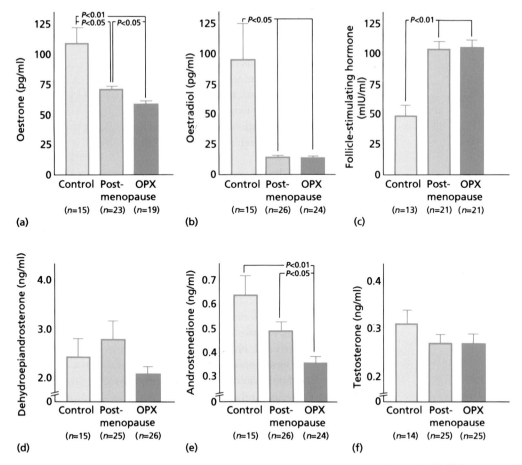

Fig. 3.7 Values for oestrogens (a and b), a gonadotrophin (follicle-stimulating hormone) (c) and some androgens (d–f) in women matched for age and weight according to menopausal status. Postmenopausal women were additionally matched for the duration of hypo-oestrogenism with subjects undergoing oophorectomy (OPX). (From Ohta *et al.*, 1992.)

duction of oestrone also declines but by less, since the peripheral aromatization of adrenal androstenedione to oestrone continues.

Indeed oestrone becomes the predominant oestrogen after the menopause. This conversion occurs largely in fat tissue so that postmenopausal oestrogenic status is dependent on fat mass (Fig. 3.8). This may explain why thinness is a risk factor for osteoporotic fracture, although there are other possible explanations.

The ovaries are also a source of androstenedione, the production of which declines after the menopause (see Table 3.3). As would be expected, androstenedione levels are lower after a surgical menopause than after a natural menopause. However, the adrenals are also a significant source of androstenedione, so that after the menopause levels fall to about 60% of those in the premenopausal state. The fall in serum testosterone is even less since the ovaries continue to secrete testosterone. Indeed, the production is increased, and the decline in serum testosterone is attributable to a decrease in its adrenal production. Oestrogen also stimulates the hepatic synthesis of sex hormone-binding globulin, which binds circulating testosterone. Thus in oestrogen deficiency the free fraction of testosterone is increased.

Since oestrogen levels decrease markedly after the menopause, it is plausible that androgens assume a more critical importance in maintaining skeletal metabolism after the menopause. Population studies have variously suggested low or normal levels of androstenedione or its precursor in osteoporotic women. Need has reported a significant correlation between residual serum dehydroepiandrosterone and bone formation rates assessed by quantitative histology in postmenopausal women with osteoporosis (Need *et al.*, 1990).

Effects of oestrogen deficiency

The menopause is a normal physiological event and not therefore a 'disease'. Irrespective of whether it is viewed as a disease, accident or physiological process, oestrogen deficiency is clearly a significant factor in the pathophysiology of many important diseases including cardiovascular disease and osteoporosis. The increased life expectancy of women in society means that these age-dependent consequences assume a progressively greater importance and justify in this context the 'medicalization of the menopause'.

A large number of clinical features have been associated with the menopause, which collectively constitute the menopausal syndrome (Table 3A). The menopause may be associated with many changes in the lifestyle of women so that not all the associations described are causal. For example, some psychological symptoms may be related to external factors such as children leaving home, divorce or death in the family. Others may be secondary to menopause-specific events such as insomnia or irritability arising from vasomotor symptoms. Psychiatric morbidity increases at the time of the menopause (Ballinger, 1975), but is not associated with an increase in depression (Jenkins & Clare, 1985). Psychiatric disorders are thus considered to be consequences of associated factors rather than causally related to oestrogen deficiency.

Hot flushes (flashes in the United States) are characteristic symptoms of oestrogen withdrawal. They are characterized by episodic sensations of warmth in the neck, face and/or upper body and typically last for several minutes. The frequency is quite variable, ranging from weekly to several times per hour. They may be associated with palpitations, an increase in heart rate, weakness and dizzi-

Testosterone

Hot flushes

Table 3.3 Changes in the pattern of hormone production after the menopause. Major changes include: a marked decrease in oestradiol production so that oestrone becomes the predominant oestrogen; and increased ovarian production of testosterone so that the ratio of androgen to oestrogen activity is increased

Hormone	Serum concentration (pmol/l)*	Source	Effects of menopause	Postmenopausal concentration (pmol/l)
Oestradiol*	240−2400	Ovary (90%) Adipose tissue (10%)	Marked decline in ovarian source	40−80
Testosterone	550−1800	Ovary (50%) Adrenal (50%)	Secretion increased Moderate reduction	520−1700
Androstenedione	2400−8900	Ovary (50%) Adrenal (50%)	Marked decrease Unchanged	800−4800
Oestrone	160−660	Adipose tissue Ovary	Decreased to 30% due to decrease in androstenedione	40−2500

* Follicular phase.

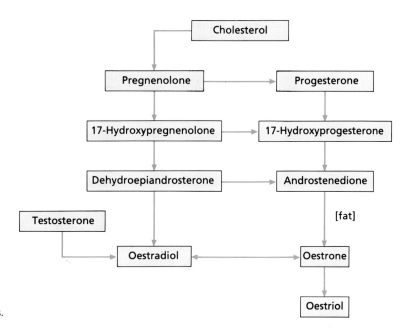

Fig. 3.8 Metabolic pathways for the synthesis of oestrogens.

ness and a visible flush which generally occurs shortly after the onset of symptoms due to an increase in peripheral blood flow. It is associated with a 1°C drop in core temperature and this results in peripheral vasodilation, increased sweating and heat loss. Hot flushes occur at any time and may wake patients from sleep giving rise to secondary symptoms such as insomnia, irritability and inability to

Table 3A Changes associated with oestrogen deficiency at the menopause

Psychological	(Not specific for oestrogen deficiency) Mood changes, irritability, lethargy and fatigue Loss of concentration Emotional lability
Urogenital	Loss of libido Vaginal atrophy, dyspareunia Urethral syndrome
Vasomotor	Hot flushes, night sweats, palpitations, insomnia
Skin	Thinning of dermis
Cardiovascular	Atherogenic lipid profile Increased risk of cardiovascular disease
Musculoskeletal	Acceleration of bone turnover and bone loss Joint pains Fractures Increase in weight and fat mass Exacerbation of rheumatoid arthritis

the suppression of bone formation. Their administration causes rapid decreases in indirect indices of skeletal metabolism, such as alkaline phosphatase and osteocalcin, and a decrease in the function of osteoblasts. The pathogenesis for this effect is far from clear and the relative contributions of altered intestinal absorption of calcium, changes in PTH and renal metabolism to diminished bone formation and increased resorption of bone are not well defined.

Intestinal absorption of calcium is decreased but the mechanism is uncertain. This is unlikely to be mediated, at least in the short term, by changes in vitamin D metabolism. Some studies have suggested that the degradation of calcidiol is increased but a more consistent observation is that neither calcidiol nor calcitriol levels decrease (Gennari et al., 1983). The mechanism is likely to be a direct effect on calcium transport, perhaps by impairing tissue sensitivity to calcitriol.

PTH

Several studies suggest that the secretion of PTH is increased in patients taking corticosteroids. Decreased intestinal absorption of calcium and perhaps decreased renal tubular reabsorption of calcium are thought to be the mechanism for the stimulation of PTH. The administration of glucocorticoids results in an increase in PTH within an hour and is not associated with measurable changes in serum calcium or calcitriol. The longer term changes in PTH metabolism are more variable. Some studies have found that most patients have high PTH values whereas others found this to be a rare phenomenon. Prospective studies suggest that marked changes in PTH secretion do not occur over an interval of several months (Prummel et al., 1991). Irrespective of whether PTH levels are high or normal with long-term treatment, there is some doubt whether this accounts for increased bone resorption (see Chapter 4).

Bone loss

The administration of glucocorticoids may also suppress the secretion of gonadotrophin-releasing hormone and adrenal production of androstenedione. In addition, they have a catabolic effect on muscle mass. All these effects may contribute to bone loss.

PTHrP

Function

PTHrP shares several homologies with PTH. Its physiological role is not yet known, but one of its functions may be the placental transport of calcium (dePapp & Stewart, 1993). It is capable of activating PTH receptors, and in many test systems, has equimolar potency. It is normally expressed in several tissues including the epidermis. High concentrations are found in lactating breast tissue, but it does not circulate systemically in health. In contrast, it is produced by a number of neoplasms and secreted into the circulation, where it is largely responsible for the humoral hypercalcaemia of malignancy. High circulating levels may contribute to generalized osteoporosis in solid tumours and, more arguably, in myelomatosis.

References

Azria M (1989) In *The Calcitonins*. Karger, Basel.

Ballinger CB (1975) Psychiatric morbidity and the menopause; screening of a general population sample. *BMJ*; **iii**: 344−346.

Bordier P, Miravet L, Matrajt H, Hioco D, Ryckewaert A (1967) Bone changes in adult patients with abnormal thyroid function (with special reference to ^{45}Ca kinetics and quantitative histology). *Proc R Soc Med*; **60**: 1132−1134.

Brincat M, Moniz CJ, Kabalan S (1987) Decline in skin collagen content and metacarpal index after the menopause and its prevention with sex hormone replacement. *Br J Obstet Gynaecol*; **94**: 126−129.

Chambers TJ, Magnus CJ (1982) Calcitonin alters behaviour of isolated osteoclasts. *J Pathol*; **82**: 27−39.

Charles P (1989) Metabolic bone disease evaluated by a combined calcium balance and tracer kinetic study. *Dan Med Bull*; **36**: 463−478.

DeLuca HF (1990) Osteoporosis and the metabolites of vitamin D. *Metabolism*; **4** (suppl. 1): 3−9.

Fitzpatrick LA, Coleman DT, Bilezikian JP (1992) The target tissue actions of parathyroid hormone. In Coe FL, Fauus MJ (eds). *Disorders of Bone and Mineral Metabolism*, pp. 123−148. Raven Press, New York.

Francis RM, Peacock M, Aaron JE *et al.* (1986) Osteoporosis in hypogonadal men: role of decreased plasma 1,25-dihydroxyvitamin D, calcium malabsorption and low bone formation. *Bone*; **7**: 261−268.

Gallagher JC, Riggs BL, Eisman J, Hamstra A, Arnaud SB, DeLuca HF (1979) Intestinal calcium absorption and serum vitamin D metabolites in normal subjects and osteoporosis patients: effect of age and dietary calcium. *J Clin Invest*; **64**: 729−736.

Gennari C, Bernini M, Nardi P *et al.* (1983) Glucocorticoids: radiocalcium and radiophosphate absorption in man. In Dixon ASJ, Russell RGG, Stamp TCB (eds). *Osteoporosis, a Multidisciplinary Problem*, pp. 75−80. Academic Press, London.

Goecke H (1959) Die Klinik des Klimakteriums. *Arch Gynak*; **193**: 33−49.

Henry HL, Norman AW (1992) Metabolism of vitamin D. In Coe FL, Favus MJ (eds). *Disorders of Bone and Mineral Metabolism*, pp. 149−193. Raven Press, New York.

Hesch R, Busch V, Prokop M, Delling G, Rittinghaus E (1989) Increase in vertebral density by combination therapy with pulsatile 1−38 hPTH and sequential addition of calcitonin nasal spray in osteoporotic patients. *Calcif Tissue Int*; **44**: 176−180.

Jenkins R, Clare AW (1985) Women and mental illness. *BMJ*; **291**: 1523−1524.

Kanis JA, Guilland-Cumming DF, Russell RGG (1982) Comparative physiology and pharmacology of the metabolites and analogues of vitamin D. In Paterson JA (ed.). *The Endocrinology of Calcium Metabolism*, pp. 321−62. Raven Press, New York.

Kleeman CR, Bohannan J, Bernstein D, Ling S, Maxwell MH (1964) Effect of variation in sodium intake on calcium excretion in normal humans. *Proc Soc Exp Biol Med*; **115**: 29−32.

Lips P, van Ginkel FC, Netelenbos JC, Wiersinga A, van der Vijgh WJ (1990) Lower mobility and markers of bone resorption in the elderly. *Bone Miner*; **9**: 45−57.

Marshall RW (1976) Plasma fractions. In Nordin BEC (ed.). *Calcium, Phosphate and Magnesium Metabolism*, pp. 162−168. Churchill Livingstone, Edinburgh.

Need AG, Durbridge TC, Nordin BEC (1990) Anabolic steroids. In Kanis JA (ed.). *Calcium Metabolism*, pp. 165−182. Karger, Basel.

Ohta H, Masuzawa T, Ikeda T, Sada Y, Makita K, Nozawa S (1992) Which is more osteoporosis-inducing, menopause or oophorectomy? *Bone Miner*; **19**: 273–285.

dePapp AE, Stewart AF (1993) Parathyroid hormone related protein. A peptide of diverse physiologic functions. *Trends Endocrinol Metab*; **4**: 181–187.

Peacock M, Nordin BEC (1968) Tubular reabsorption of calcium in normal and hypercalciuric subjects. *J Clin Pathol*; **21**: 353–358.

Prummel MF, Wiersinga WM, Lips P, Sanders GTB, Sauerwein HP (1991) The course of biochemical parameters of bone turnover during treatment with corticosteroids. *J Clin Endocrinol*; **72**: 382–386.

Reginster J, Deroisy R, Albert A *et al.* (1989) Relationship between whole plasma calcitonin levels, calcitonin secretory capacity, and plasma levels of estrone in healthy women and postmenopausal osteoporotics. *J Clin Invest*; **83**: 1073–1077.

Selby PL, Peacock M (1986) Ethinyloestradiol and norethisterone in the treatment of primary hyperparathyroidism in postmenopausal women. *N Engl J Med*; **314**: 1481–1485.

Sokoll LJ, Morrow FD, Quirbach DM, Dawson-Hughes B (1988) Intact parathyrin in postmenopausal women. *Clin Chem*; **34**: 407–410.

Staub JF, Tracqui P, Lausson S, Milhaud G, Perault-Staub AM (1989) A physiological view of *in vivo* calcium dynamics: the regulation of a nonlinear self-organised system. *Bone*; **10**: 77–86.

Stock JL, Coderre JA, Posillico JT (1988) Effects of estrogen on mineral metabolism in postmenopausal women as evaluated by multiple assays measuring parathyroid hormone bioactivity. *J Bone Miner Res*; **2** (suppl.) S161.

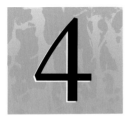

Causes of osteoporosis

Bone mass of an individual is a function of peak bone mass and subsequent losses. Since osteoporosis may arise from abnormalities at all stages of skeletal life, it is difficult to provide an accurate classification of osteoporosis. Rather, it may be more useful to consider osteoporosis as predominantly multifactorial and to describe the factors and their relative importance. For example, factors such as age, sex and disease are important determinants of bone mass and fracture, as well as lifestyle influences including diet, exercise and smoking.

Multifactorial

Hypogonadal bone loss

By far the most common cause of hypogonadal osteoporosis is that associated with the natural menopause, but all causes of gonadal insufficiency induce bone loss and many have been associated with an increase in the risk of osteoporotic fractures (Table 4A). Hysterectomy with bilateral oophorectomy induces marked loss of bone and initial rates of loss exceed those occurring in women undergoing a natural menopause, but there is little evidence that the ultimate losses are increased over and above that expected from an early menopause (Ohta *et al.*, 1992). Hysterectomy without oophorectomy may induce a temporary cessation of ovarian function, presumably related to interference with the ovarian blood supply. In some cases this may be irreversible. There is some evidence that the onset of the menopause may be accelerated by simple hysterectomy and even by tubal ligation, and in view of the high frequency of hysterectomy in many countries it has been considered that such women should be identified and assessed for their risk of osteoporosis.

Simple hysterectomy

Men do not undergo an abrupt menopause in the same way as women, though androgen status declines in some elderly men. Whereas this might contribute to skeletal losses, the relationship between declining gonadal status and risk of fracture in men has not been fully explored. Overt hypogonadism is an important cause of osteoporosis in men and gives rise to fractures. The histological findings are comparable to those found in oestrogen deficiency in

Hypogonadism in men

Table 4A Some causes of hypogonadal osteoporosis

In women
Natural menopause, especially if early
Bilateral oophorectomy
Hysterectomy and tubal ligation
Late menarche
Anorexia nervosa and other causes of weight loss
Exercise-induced amenorrhoea
Chemotherapy

In men
Eunuchoidism
Orchiectomy
Klinefelter's syndrome
Kallmann's syndrome
Prepubertal castration syndrome
Delayed puberty

In men and women
Haemochromatosis
Chronic malnutrition
Gonadal dysgenesis
Gonadotrophin-releasing hormone analogues
Chronic liver disease
Gonadal irradiation
Pituitary disease (with gonadal insufficiency)

women and include the disruption of skeletal architecture (Francis *et al.*, 1986). Causes in men include castration, for example after prostatic surgery, hypopituitarism, Klinefelter's syndrome and other diseases and drugs that impair gonadal function in women.

Involutional bone loss

'Age-related' loss

The term involutional or 'age-related' bone loss describes the continued bone loss that occurs in men and therefore is assumed to occur in women throughout later life. The evidence for age-related bone loss in humans is largely drawn from population studies which may underestimate the rate of loss. Adjustment of bone mass for muscle mass all but eliminates the apparent loss, suggesting that skeletal mass remains appropriate for muscle mass. The extent to which this accounts for age-related losses is unknown and will depend upon the outcome of adequately designed prospective studies. Since muscle mass also declines in women with advancing age, it

Decreased muscle mass

would be expected that age-related losses should also occur due to a similar phenomenon. Indeed, adjustment for muscle mass (e.g., total body potassium) decreases the apparent loss with age in population studies (Thomsen *et al.*, 1986).

Nutritional causes of osteoporosis

Many nutritional causes of osteoporosis have been proposed (Table 4B) but in many instances the association may be fortuitous. The more important causes are reviewed below.

CALCIUM

There is no compelling evidence to suggest that on a mixed diet calcium plays a critical role in the attainment of peak bone mass. Small differences in apparent skeletal density account for differences in remodelling space (see Chapter 2). In contrast, changes in bone remodelling are likely to have a greater consequence when superimposed on a bone losing state.

> Since oestrogen deficiency induces a focal imbalance at remodelling sites, metabolic changes which increase the remodelling rate of bone will accelerate skeletal losses still further. The effect of a low dietary intake of calcium in osteoporosis appears to be due to an increase in bone turnover.

Thus skeletal losses after the menopause can be accelerated by low calcium diets and pharmacological doses of calcium can delay the rate of bone loss (see Chapter 7). It has been argued that osteoporosis is a calcium-deficiency disorder (Nordin & Morris, 1989). Reduced calcium absorption, low values for calcitriol and target tissue resistance to calcitriol have also been used as arguments, but views differ depending on whether these abnormalities are considered as causes or consequences of postmenopausal osteoporosis (see Chapter 3). A further argument in favour of considering osteoporosis as a calcium-deficiency syndrome is that studies of calcium requirements suggest that these are increased in osteoporosis using balance techniques, but none may be interpreted with confidence (see Chapter 2).

Table 4B Some nutritional factors that have been associated with an increased risk of osteoporosis

Low calcium intake*
Low intake of vitamin D*
Malnutrition
High protein or phosphate diet
Caffeine
High sodium diet
High intake of alcohol
Low intake of fluoride*
Vitamin K deficiency
Scurvy
Vitamin B_6 and B_{12} deficiency
Zinc and boron deficiency

* See also Chapter 2.

It is also evident that differences in calcium nutrition around the world cannot explain differences in the risk of fractures between communities.

> Hip fractures occur commonly in those communities with higher intakes of calcium, such as Scandinavia and Holland, whereas hip fracture rates are lower in those communities with lower dietary intakes (see Chapter 2). This should not be interpreted to mean that calcium cannot modify the natural history of osteoporosis, nor that a high calcium intake causes osteoporosis – only that differences in calcium nutrition cannot explain the marked differences in fracture risk between communities.

These various observations suggest that osteoporosis is not a disease due to calcium deficiency. Although skeletal calcium losses are clearly attenuated by the pharmacological manipulation of bone turnover, this argues that calcium deficiency causes osteoporosis only in the same sense that penicillin deficiency causes streptococcal infections.

Pharmacological interventions

It is perhaps more appropriate to consider both calcium and penicillin to be pharmacological interventions rather than related to the causes of disease.

VITAMIN D

Prolonged vitamin D deficiency induces osteomalacia which may complicate osteoporosis. Progressive hypomineralization of bone decreases its mechanical competence and increases the risk of fracture. The features of less marked deficiency, or vitamin D deficiency of a shorter duration, include secondary hyperparathyroidism and an increase in the activation frequency of bone. As in the case of a low calcium diet, this would be expected to accelerate bone loss.

Aging and vitamin D

> Although disturbances in vitamin D metabolism have been observed in association with the menopause, the balance of evidence would suggest that they are a consequence of osteoporosis rather than a contributing factor. There is more evidence that disturbances in vitamin D metabolism occur with aging due to the decline in renal function causing secondary hyperparathyroidism (see Chapter 3). There is no clear evidence that these abnormalities are associated with osteoporosis but this is plausible.

Cause of fracture

The question arises how often secondary hyperparathyroidism is complicated by privational deficiency of vitamin D and if so whether it contributes to fracture risk. Vitamin D deficiency is a well-recognized cause of fracture. The frequency with which it occurs is more difficult to judge because the distinction between hyperparathyroid bone disease and mild vitamin D deficiency is not straightforward (see Chapter 2) and the results of many histological studies in patients with hip fracture which have reported a high prevalence of osteomalacia do not make this distinction. Where the distinction is made, for example by measuring the osteoid seam width, this has been shown to be normal (Lips *et al.*, 1982) or increased (Hordon & Peacock, 1990). A further problem is that the sensitivity and specificity of calcidiol measurements as an index of osteomalacia are poor. For example, the normal range for the young healthy adult in the United Kingdom would be regarded as pathologically low in the United States. Moreover, though calcidiol values are lower than controls in some series of hip fracture (Lips *et al.*, 1982), this is by no means an invariant finding.

Vitamin D-induced osteomalacia

Nevertheless, there is good evidence that vitamin D-induced osteomalacia does occur and contributes to fracture in a minority. Osteomalacia due to vitamin D deficiency is well recognized to occur in the elderly, in institutions or geriatric hospitals where exposure to sunlight is low and nutrition may be borderline. In addition, the age- and sex-specific risk of hip and other fractures is high in such communities. The reasons for impaired nutritional status of vitamin D in the elderly are multifactorial. Major factors include dietary deficiency and lack of exposure to sunlight. Other factors proposed have been a decrease in the synthetic capacity of the skin to convert 7-dehydrocholesterol but there is little evidence for this view. In such patients, the use of vitamin D and calcium may decrease the risk of hip and other osteoporotic fractures (see Chapter 9).

PROTEIN AND PHOSPHATE

Childhood deficiency

Marked protein calorie malnutrition and prolonged vitamin D deficiency during childhood have a significant effect on skeletal development and the bone mass attained. The impact of this on subsequent fracture risk is not known, but is plausible since this delays puberty which is well established as a risk. The effects of more modest dietary perturbations are not really known, but it is possible that malnutrition may be an important factor in the elderly. Patients with hip fracture are generally less well nourished than their age-matched controls, and malnutrition is associated with an

Undernutrition

increased risk of falling. Undernutrition is often reported in the elderly and may contribute to bone loss, the risk of falling or the response to injury. In patients with hip fracture attention to nutrition during the hospital stay decreases the risk of complications and mortality (Delmi *et al.*, 1990).

In contrast, several studies have suggested that a high intake of protein might increase the risk of osteoporosis. The administration of animal protein may induce calciuria. The steady-state changes have, however, not been explored. There are ecological correlates with protein intake and hip fracture risk, but the causal relationship is far from certain.

High phosphate diets may induce secondary hyperparathyroidism and hypercalciuria. The mechanism for the increases in urinary calcium may be similar to that observed following the high intake of protein. It should be noted that the increase in the urinary excretion of calcium has been observed over relatively short intervals after dietary manipulation and may not reflect steady-state changes. Moreover, changes in bone remodelling are unlikely to affect peak bone mass other than for this reason. The relevance of these dietary indiscretions if any to osteoporosis is not known.

CAFFEINE

Coffee and tea

High intakes of caffeine have been recorded in patients with osteoporosis in some but not all studies. The administration of caffeine-containing drinks can increase the urinary excretion rate for calcium (Heaney & Recker, 1982). As in the case for high protein loads, the relevance of this to peak bone mass is questionable. With respect to its contribution to osteoporosis, the data are at best circumstantial and not convincing. There have been cohort studies noting an association between coffee consumption and the risk of hip fracture, but these are not consistent. Moreover, tea which also contains caffeine, appears to be associated with a decrease in hip fracture risk, perhaps related to the presence of oestrogenic flavinoids.

SODIUM INTAKE

High sodium diets have been shown to increase the urinary excretion of calcium in experimental animals and, in humans, this is associated with an increase in biochemical indices of bone turnover including increased urinary excretion of hydroxyproline. This is most likely due to a decrease in renal tubular reabsorption of calcium which would suggest that the lower serum calcium thereby induced might stimulate the secretion of parathyroid hormone (PTH) and increase the activation frequency of bone. Population studies have shown an association between sodium and calcium excretion but the steady-state effects of a high sodium diet have not been reported (Goulding, 1981). If persistent, it could however accelerate losses in a situation where a patient was not otherwise in balance for calcium.

ALCOHOL

Dietary disturbances

Alcohol abuse appears to be a significant risk factor for osteoporosis particularly in men. Reduced rates of bone formation have been reported to be associated with ethanol consumption in humans and experimental animals. A high intake of alcohol is associated with marked dietary disturbances such as protein undernutrition, other changes in lifestyle, liver disease and a decrease in testosterone which may have additional effects. In one study (Diamond *et al.*, 1989) a 'control' group comprised of alcoholics who had abstained from alcohol differed little from the test group in most characteristics except that bone formation rates were markedly decreased (Table 4.1).

Table 4.1 Histological findings (mean ± SEM) in patients with alcoholic liver disease divided according to their current consumption of alcohol. (From Diamond et al., 1989)

	Controls (n = 35)	Abstainers (n = 12)	Drinkers (n = 28)
Bone volume (% tissue volume)	24.2 ± 0.5	19.6 ± 0.7*	20.6 ± 0.8*
Osteoid volume (% bone volume)	2.2 ± 0.2	2.1 ± 0.3	1.4 ± 0.1*†
Osteoid surface (% bone surface)	12.1 ± 0.6	10.2 ± 1.2	7.0 ± 0.6*†
Osteoid width (μm)	11.1 ± 0.3	10.2 ± 0.6*	8.7 ± 0.3*
Osteoblast surface (% bone surface)	4.7 ± 0.4	3.8 ± 0.5	1.8 ± 0.3*†
Osteoclast surface (% bone surface)	1.5 ± 0.1	1.6 ± 0.3	1.3 ± 0.3
Bone formation rate ($\mu m^3/\mu m^2$/day)	6 ± 1	5 ± 1	1 ± 1*†

* Significantly lower than control values.
† Significantly lower than abstainers.

OTHER DIETARY FACTORS

A host of other factors have been associated with bone mass in ecological studies. These include the dietary intake of zinc, vitamin B_{12}, boron and vitamin K, vitamin B_6, silicon and vitamin C. Vitamins C and B_6 are both cofactors for normal collagen metabolism and overt deficiencies of either may give rise to osteoporosis.

Other endocrine causes of osteoporosis

Apart from gonadal deficiency a number of other endocrine diseases are also associated with osteoporosis, though their occurrence in the general population is in many instances relatively low. They are, however, important to identify since specific treatment will in some instances modify the osteoporotic process.

PRIMARY HYPERPARATHYROIDISM

Primary hyperparathyroidism is common and affects approximately one in 1000 of the general population. In the majority (85%), hypercalcaemia is associated with the presence of a single chief cell adenoma in one of the four parathyroid glands. It most commonly occurs in women and presents shortly after the menopause. This suggests that oestrogen and/or progestogen withdrawal is a contributory factor to its development or expression. Indeed, hormone replacement therapy (HRT) may lower serum calcium levels in postmenopausal women with hyperparathyroidism (Selby & Peacock, 1986). It is not known

Common in postmenopausal women

whether this is due to an effect of gonadal steroids on PTH secretion or on bone (see Chapter 3).

The effects of primary hyperparathyroidism on bone are to increase the activation frequency of bone remodelling. Thus, all elements of bone turnover are increased and these decrease following parathyroid surgery (Christiansen *et al.*, 1990). The effects on bone mass are consistent with that expected from an increased turnover. Histomorphometric studies have shown a reduction in cancellous bone volume as has absorptiometry at appendicular and axial sites. There is indirect evidence that connectivity of cancellous bone is preserved implying that bone strength might be restored if bone mass were to be increased. This may be true as a generalization but prospective studies show that the increment in bone mass after parathyroidectomy is transient over 1 year, that remaining deficits are not regained thereafter and that patients may remain osteoporotic, at least at the wrist.

Clinical features

A large proportion of patients with primary hyperparathyroidism are detected by routine blood analyses, and are relatively asymptomatic. When symptoms are present, these are usually due to hypercalcaemia. Bone pain is an uncommon presentation of primary hyperparathyroidism in all but the most severe cases. Radiographic features include subperiosteal erosions classically seen on the radial borders of the middle phalanges, the distal ends of the clavicles and bone resorption in the skull (resulting in a mottled or 'salt and pepper' appearance), but occur in less than 2% of patients. Fractures are also well-recognized problems of severe hyperparathyroidism. The controversy arises over the risks in mildly affected patients, particularly in postmenopausal women, since many would manage such patients conservatively. An increase in the risk of vertebral fractures has been shown in several population studies (Fig. 4.1). A more recent study showed no increase in risk and questioned the adequacy of the controls used in other studies.

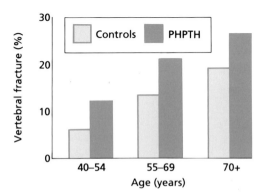

Fig. 4.1 Prevalence of vertebral compression fractures in 191 patients with primary hyperparathyroidism (PTPTH) aged 40 years or more compared with that in age-matched patients referred for cholecystectomy. None was referred for bone disease. (From Kochersberger *et al.*, 1987.)

Diagnosis and treatment

In the majority of patients, the diagnosis of primary hyperparathyroidism is straightforward and depends on the finding of an inappropriately high circulating level of PTH in the presence of hypercalcaemia. In the interpretation of values of PTH, the effect of impairment of renal function on the assay results needs to be taken into account, particularly if region-specific assays are utilized.

Assays

The treatment of choice in most patients with primary hyperparathyroidism is neck exploration and excision of the adenoma. Conservative management is advocated by some in elderly patients with mild, uncomplicated hypercalcaemia. Medical management has its limitations. Gonadal steroids and androgenic progestogens (e.g., norethisterone 5 mg daily) may be of value in postmenopausal women who refuse surgery or who pose too great an operative risk (Selby & Peacock, 1986). The bisphosphonates can probably prevent progressive bone loss, but the effects on serum calcium are relatively short lived (months) (Hamdy et al., 1987).

Medical treatment

In an asymptomatic patient with osteoporosis and hyperparathyroidism the options for treatment are not straightforward. Some would argue that patients should be merely followed because mild hyperparathyroidism is not associated with accelerated osteoporosis and surgery is meddlesome. On the other hand, constant review of patients is meddlesome and for this reason many err on the side of surgery.

THYROTOXICOSIS

Osteoporosis occurs in long-standing hyperthyroidism. Patients with hyperthyroidism show an increase in the rate of bone remodelling and biochemical indices of bone turnover may be increased moderately. Hypercalciuria is common but hypercalcaemia occurs rarely. The mechanism is thought to be due to a direct action of thyroid hormone to increase bone turnover (see Chapter 3).

It is to be expected that in later life, where bone loss is occurring in men or women, thyrotoxicosis would accelerate these losses. Elderly patients may have relatively few physical signs of thyrotoxicosis so that the diagnosis may be missed. For this reason, many incorporate measurements of thyroid hormones or thyroid-stimulating hormone (TSH) in the evaluation of elderly patients with osteoporosis.

Occult disease

Another important cause for thyroid bone disease is the improper use of long-term thyroid replacement therapy (see below).

CUSHING'S SYNDROME

The adverse effects of glucocorticoids on skeletal metabolism are well established and were first described by Cushing in 1932. Cushing's syndrome is associated with progressive osteoporosis and fractures. Osteoporosis is said to be more marked at axial than appendicular

Associations

sites, but the evidence for this in long-standing Cushing's syndrome is wanting. Occasionally, Cushing's syndrome may present with osteoporosis and the diagnosis only becomes evident after further investigation. More usually it is associated with other features of Cushing's syndrome such as hypertension, centripedal obesity, atrophic changes in the skin and diabetes mellitus.

> The mechanism of action of glucocorticosteroids is complex (see Chapter 3), but the features in bone have been well described. These are discussed subsequently (see Drugs causing osteoporosis).

INSULIN-DEPENDENT DIABETES MELLITUS

Reduced bone mineral content has been observed in several studies examining the risk of osteoporosis in diabetes, which may be less marked at cancellous bone sites. In individual cases radiographic changes may be marked. Some studies suggest that osteoporosis is more marked in those with poorly controlled diabetes. There are several reports of fractures occurring associated with diabetes. A large case-control study from Rochester did not show any increase in the risk of fractures in long-standing insulin-dependent diabetics (Heath *et al.*, 1980), though the adequacy of the control population has been questioned. Indeed a decreased risk was observed at some sites. There is, therefore, a disparity between the densitometric studies and studies of fracture rates.

Peripheral neuropathy

> The densitometric measurements may be inaccurate because of changes in body composition in diabetics. Additionally, an increased risk of fracture may be confined to a subpopulation of diabetic patients. An increased risk of fracture has been noted in those with peripheral neuropathy where cortical osteoporosis may be marked, and a high incidence of ankle fractures was recorded in the Rochester study of fracture risk (Heath *et al.*, 1980).

Drugs causing osteoporosis

Many drugs affect skeletal metabolism (Table 4C). Others have been thought, on the basis of short-term investigations or animal experiments, to affect skeletal metabolism adversely. These include theophyllines, the phenothiazines, nitrites, calcium channel blockers and cyclosporin A. Their relevance to osteoporosis is not known.

SMOKING

There are many reasons to advise individuals to stop smoking particularly in relation to lung cancer and chronic respiratory disease.

Table 4C Drugs associated with an increased risk of osteoporosis

Smoking
Glucocorticosteroids and adrenocorticotrophin
Thyroxine
Anticonvulsants
Heparin
Lithium
Cytotoxic drugs
Gonadotrophin-releasing hormone agonists
Tamoxifen (premenopausal use)
Aluminium
Vitamin D
Drugs causing falls
Hyperoxia

Many believe that the risk of osteoporosis is also increased in smokers but the evidence for this is circumstantial and largely based on epidemiological correlates.

There are several reasons for considering smoking as a risk factor (Table 4D). Smokers are generally thinner than their non-smoking counterparts which may in part account for the risk. Since an important source of oestrogen in the postmenopausal woman is in adipose tissue, the decrease in fat mass may increase this risk. There is however also evidence that smoking might increase the catabolism of oestradiol. The hepatic metabolism of oestradiol to the 2-hydroxy derivatives of low biological activity is increased. Smoking may also accelerate the metabolism of exogenous oestrogen and induce an earlier menopause. The increased risk of osteoporosis associated with a low body mass may not be solely related to the postmenopausal production of oestrogen, but may be due to decreased weight on the skeleton. Finally, smokers differ from their non-smoking counterparts in several important respects including a higher consumption of alcohol and a lower degree of physical activity.

Induced weight loss

Earlier menopause

CORTICOSTEROIDS

The exogenous use of corticosteroids and adrenocorticotrophin has

Table 4D Putative effects of smoking in relationship to osteoporosis

Accelerated menopause
Decreased fat mass
Decreased peripheral production of oestrogen
Decreased resistance to falls
Decreased weight on skeleton
Accelerated metabolism of endogenous oestrogen
Accelerated metabolism of exogenous oestrogens
Association with alcohol consumption and other lifestyle factors

been recognized as a risk factor since the 1940s. Many studies have shown a decrease in bone mass and an increase in the risk of fractures particularly those of the ribs and of the wrist which have occurred in 30–50% of populations studied (Reid, 1989).

The manner in which glucocorticoids induce bone loss is complex (Fig. 4.2; see Chapter 3). One of the problems is that there are difficulties interpreting some of the effects of glucocorticoids *in vitro* and also in experimental animals. For example, glucocorticoids may increase bone mineral in some animals. The administration of glucocorticoids may also suppress the adrenal production of androstenedione and in this way may accelerate postmenopausal losses. In addition, corticosteroids have a catabolic effect on muscle mass and this in turn may adversely affect skeletal metabolism.

Androstenedione

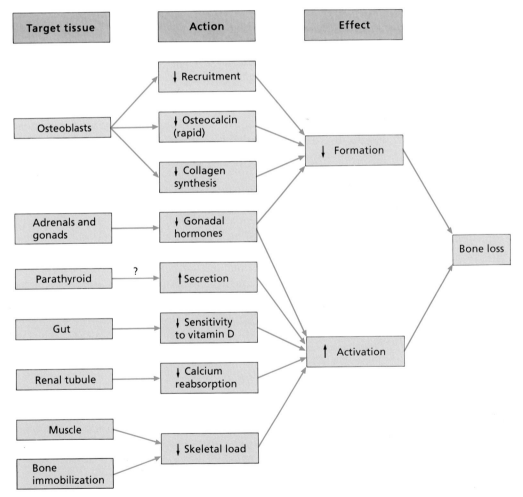

Fig. 4.2 Simplified schema to illustrate effects of excess glucocorticoids on skeletal metabolism.

In the assessment of skeletal status, it is important to recall that steroids induce changes in body composition and in the ratio of fat to lean body mass. This may introduce systematic inaccuracies in the estimation of bone mineral. In humans the assessment is complicated by the underlying disease state, the wide range of doses used and concurrent drugs affecting bone metabolism and immobilization.

Most clinical research suggests that glucocorticoids have a direct effect on osteoblast function. The acute administration of glucocorticoids results in the suppression of osteoblast markers such as alkaline phosphatase and osteocalcin (Reid, 1989). Over a longer period the wall thickness of newly completed bone remodelling units is reduced by 25% (Bressot et al., 1979) indicating a decreased amount of bone deposited within each erosion cavity.

The mineral apposition rate (MAR) is markedly impaired to approximately 50% of control values and accounts for the decrease in bone formation. This results in a progressive decrease in bone mineral with time and may be exacerbated by other factors which accelerate bone loss such as the menopause, the underlying disease and immobilization. Indeed, rates of bone loss have been shown to be accelerated in postmenopausal women taking corticosteroids compared to their premenopausal counterparts.

Some but not all studies suggest that PTH secretion is increased. Similarly, some but not all show increased resorption on bone biopsy. Neither is there a clear relationship between the two. This suggests that a degree of hyperparathyroidism may complicate glucocorticoid-induced osteoporosis in some patients. The expression of hyperparathyroidism may relate to, on the one hand, an effect of steroids to increase PTH secretion and, on the other hand, an effect of skeletal calcium losses to decrease this. In some cases, increased bone resorption may be the result of the immobilization associated with chronic disease. Another factor is that corticosteroids affect the secretion and metabolism of gonadal steroids which would increase bone resorption.

Many studies have documented the loss of bone at all sites accessible to measurement (Fig. 4.3). Several investigators have suggested that bone loss may occur preferentially at axial rather than appendicular sites. This may only reflect the proportion of cancellous bone at the site of measurement, since losses at these sites are expected to be greater than at cortical sites. Long-term exposure therefore decreases bone mass at all sites, but vertebral fractures occur sooner than hip fractures.

There are relatively few prospective studies documenting the natural history of glucocorticoid-induced bone loss. Studies undertaken over 2 years show progressive losses at the femur and lumbar spine. The

Direct effect on osteoblasts

PTH secretion increased

Gonadal steroids

Long-term exposure

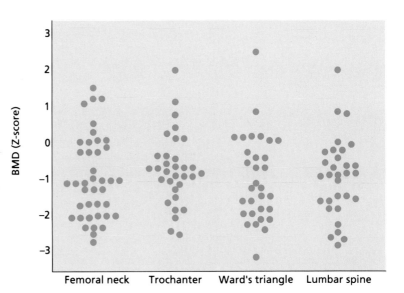

Fig. 4.3 Bone mineral density (BMD) assessed by dual photon absorptiometry at the hip and lumbar spine in patients receiving corticosteroids for an average of 6.6 years (average prednisolone dose 12.7 mg daily). (From Sambrook *et al.*, 1990.)

constant rate of change in bone density suggests an imbalance at remodelling sites without an increase in the activation frequency of bone. On the other hand, the rate of loss may decrease with time and significantly slower rates of loss are recorded in prospective studies where patients taking corticosteroids for different durations were compared (Sambrook *et al.*, 1990) or in patients followed immediately after starting treatment (Gennari & Civitelli, 1986):

Susceptibility

The susceptibility to bone loss may not be the same in all disorders for which steroids are used. Some studies have shown that younger patients are at greater risk. It is a clinical impression that many patients with end-stage chronic renal failure tolerate large doses of corticosteroids without adverse effects on skeletal mass. However, after renal, cardiac and liver transplantation skeletal losses are usually rapid. It has been difficult to demonstrate dose−response effects (Gennari & Civitelli, 1986), perhaps related to variations in susceptibility. Indeed, there is some degree of uncertainty whether low doses of glucocorticoid invariably decrease bone mass. Some studies suggest that the bone mass at the appendicular skeleton in premenopausal women is not affected by the administration of modest amounts of corticosteroids (e.g., prednisolone 7.5 mg daily). With postmenopausal women on the same dose of glucocorticoids, skeleton losses are accelerated.

Alternate-day glucocorticoid therapy appears to have a beneficial effect on growth and the suppression of the hypothalamic−pituitary−adrenal axis, but does not reduce the adverse effects on the skeleton.

Inhaled corticosteroids

It is a misconception that inhaled corticosteroids are not absorbed, though systemic absorption is markedly decreased. Their use is associated with changes in some of the indirect indices of skeletal metabolism such as serum osteocalcin, suggesting that their use might decrease bone formation.

Skeletal abnormalities

The use of glucocorticoids is associated with other skeletal abnormalities. High doses of glucocorticoids, particularly in the presence of renal failure, increase the risk of avascular necrosis. A commonly affected site is the femoral head, but it may occur at many sites. It is notable that the callus associated with fractures is slow to resolve in the glucocorticoid-treated patient, which may represent an abnormality in bone to respond appropriately to mechanical loads. This gives rise to the presence of pseudocallus which is a helpful sign in the radiographic evaluation of osteoporosis (see Chapter 5).

THYROXINE

Hypothyroidism is common particularly in postmenopausal women where the prevalence is 7% over the age of 60 years. Disturbances in calcium and bone metabolism are well described in patients with thyrotoxicosis, and might be expected to occur in some patients receiving thyroxine-replacement therapy.

Common

> Treatment of hypothyroid patients results in a decrease in bone mineral density (BMD) (Ribot *et al.*, 1990) consistent with an increase in the activation frequency of bone. Thus, losses are more marked in the first 6 months of treatment and are largely complete after 1 year. It is likely that the exuberant use of thyroid-replacement treatment contributes to additional bone loss.

Patients in whom thyroid-stimulating hormone (TSH) is suppressed using sensitive assays have accelerated losses of bone but normal rates of loss occur when thyroid function tests are kept within the normal range. In the United States, 80% of patients treated with thyroxine-replacement treatment were considered to receive excessive amounts of thyroxine, as judged by the response of TSH to thyroid-releasing hormone (TRH). This suggests that a standard dose of thyroxine is not suitable for all patients and indeed the requirements for thyroxine probably decrease with age. This has led to the widespread view that doses of thyroid hormone should be adjusted according to TSH levels. This may be somewhat evangelical since undertreatment is also not without potential long-term risks. It may therefore be appropriate to assess skeletal risk and then consider treatment for bone loss.

ANTICONVULSANTS

Osteomalacia

Anticonvulsants have long been associated with osteomalacia, but this may be due in part to the fact that many studies have been undertaken in institutionalized patients who were at high risk from vitamin D deficiency and osteomalacia. Notwithstanding, anticonvulsants are inducers of microsomal enzymes and increase the catabolism of vitamin D metabolites, particularly 25-hydroxyvitamin D. In addition, they may accelerate the catabolism of 17β-oestradiol. High doses of anticonvulsants appear to decrease calcium absorption, perhaps in part mediated by a decrease in the circulating concentration of calcidiol. A more important effect may be to decrease the target tissue responses to calcitriol. As in the case of chronic liver disease, the use of anticonvulsants is more often associated with osteoporosis than with osteomalacia.

HEPARIN

Generalized osteoporosis and spontaneous fractures occur in patients treated with heparin and are likely to be related to a direct effect on osteoclast development and activity. The doses required are substantial (10 000–15 000 U daily), most commonly used in pregnancy where warfarin is contraindicated. The extent of the reversibility of bone loss is uncertain. A radiographic survey suggested no evidence of permanent osteoporosis, but this is not adequate evidence for reversibility.

Low-molecular-weight heparins are increasingly being used in women with risk factors for clotting during pregnancy, but the effects on bone mass are not yet known.

LITHIUM

Treatment with lithium appears to increase the secretion of PTH and hypercalcaemia. Long-term treatment is associated with hyperparathyroidism, which in turn may accelerate bone loss and decreased bone mineral content is reported following its use.

CYTOTOXIC DRUGS

Cytotoxic chemotherapy has adverse effects on skeletal metabolism as well as on many other tissues. Use of such agents is therefore likely to have a direct toxic effect on bone metabolism. In addition, gonadal tissues are particularly sensitive to chemotherapy, and approximately 50% of premenopausal women receiving adjuvant chemotherapy for breast cancer will have a chemotherapy-induced menopause.

GONADOTROPHIN-RELEASING HORMONE AND LUTEINIZING HORMONE-RELEASING HORMONE ANTAGONISTS OR AGONISTS

This class of drug is being used increasingly for premenstrual syndrome, polycystic ovaries, endometriosis, breast feeding and prostatic cancer. Treatment-induced suppression of gonadal steroids results in bone loss. Although short-term treatment is associated with losses that are largely reversible (Cann et al., 1987), presumably related to the increase in bone turnover that is the early feature of gonadal insufficiency, the long-term use of these agents is likely to result in a more permanent deficit. Depot medroxyprogesterone acetate is used as a contraceptive, since it inhibits the secretion of pituitary gonado-trophins. Its use in premenopausal women lowers bone mass but appears to be reversible.

TAMOXIFEN

Protective effect

Tamoxifen is an oestrogen antagonist with weak agonist activity which is being widely used as an adjuvant in breast cancer. Its weak oestrogenic effects appear to have a protective effect on the skeleton in oestrogen-deficient women (see Chapter 6). The effect of tamoxifen in premenopausal women is not known with certainty, but it seems possible that it may induce modest decreases in BMD (Gotfredsen *et al.*, 1984). In view of the increasing use of this agent as an adjuvant it will be important to delineate the long-term effects of this agent on bone.

VITAMIN D TOXICITY AND SENSITIVITY

Skeletal toxicity

Iatrogenic vitamin D toxicity is common. It causes hypercalcaemia, hyperphosphataemia and if prolonged also induces osteoporosis. Skeletal toxicity occurs with doses of vitamin D above 10 000 IU daily. The therapeutic window is much lower with the 1α-hydroxylated derivatives of vitamin D. Where toxicity is induced with parent vitamin D or calcidiol, hypercalcaemia and osteopenia may develop many months or even years after the start of treatment and, because of their long half-life and storage in fatty tissues, reversal may take many months. Hypercalcaemia responds to treatment with corti-costeroids or bisphosphonates, which occasionally may need to be given for many months or years after treatment is stopped. The 1α-hydroxylated derivatives of vitamin D (calcitriol, alfacalcidol and dihydrotachysterol) have a more rapid onset and offset of action. Thus, patients present rapidly with hypercalcaemia and drug-induced osteoporosis is rare.

Hypercalcaemia

Serum levels of calcitriol are not markedly increased in vitamin D toxicity caused by the parent vitamin since the kidneys can regulate the production of calcitriol. In contrast, there are a number of dis-orders where the close regulation of the 1α-hydroxylase is impaired and toxicity occurs with modest challenges of vitamin D. Mild or transient hypercalcaemia occurs in approximately 10% of patients with sarcoidosis and hypercalciuria and increased bone resorption is considerably more common. Extrarenal synthesis of calcitriol also occurs more rarely in other granulomatous diseases including tubercu-losis, berylliosis, coccidioïdomycosis and histoplasmosis and in some patients with lymphoma.

Vitamin D-sensitive disorders

DRUGS AND THE RISK OF FALLING
A number of drugs have been associated with an increased risk of hip

fracture. These include alcohol, hypoglycaemic agents, minor and major tranquillizers and a range of hypnotics. It seems plausible that the use of these agents might be associated with postural hypotension or disorientation which might increase the risk of falling. Other drugs associated with hip fracture are loop diuretics and digoxin. The evidence that these increase the risk of fracture is based largely upon epidemiological surveys which show conflicting results. It seems possible that in many instances the increased risk of hip fracture relates to the comorbidity associated with drug use rather than the treatment for these associated disorders (Jensen *et al.*, 1991).

Clinical disorders associated with osteoporosis

Many other clinical disorders are associated with osteoporosis (Table 4E), the most common are reviewed below.

NEOPLASIA AFFECTING THE SKELETON

Osteoporosis is a common complication of several neoplastic disorders. Solid tumours commonly produce focal osteolytic disease but many solid tumours also induce a generalized increase in bone resorption, particularly in the case of breast cancer. Osteoclasts are stimulated by systemic factors released into the circulation by the tumour. These factors include the PTH-related peptide (PTHrP) (see Chapter 2) and more rarely PTH itself or calcitriol in human T-lymphotropic virus-associated lymphoma. There are several other reasons why women with breast cancer are at increased risk from osteoporosis. In addition to a humoral component of bone resorption, several adjuvants may directly or indirectly affect skeletal metabolism. These include the use of tamoxifen and chemotherapy (see pp. 96–97).

Generalized osteopaenia may be a presenting feature of myelomatosis (Kyle, 1975). The major mechanism for the induction of osteolysis is the activation of osteoclastic bone resorption by cytokines secreted by abnormal plasma cells. These include interleukin-6 and lymphotoxin, which increase the recruitment of osteoclast precursors to the osteoclast pool. Although chemotherapy is the mainstay of treatment of myelomatosis, it is not curative and does not heal bone lesions. Indeed, progressive bone resorption and fractures commonly occur despite apparently stable disease (Delmas *et al.*, 1982). All aspects of bone remodelling are increased, including the number of osteoblasts (Fig. 4.4). However, the functional competence of osteoblasts is impaired, as judged by the modest changes in bone formation rate. Thus, a major mechanism for bone loss is an imbalance between resorption and formation and acceleration of bone turnover. With more advanced tumour loads the eroded surface increases progressively but the number of osteoclasts is not correspondingly increased. Possible explanations include non-osteoclast-mediated resorption or uncoupling of bone formation from previous resorption.

Bone resorption

Cytokines

Table 4E Diseases associated with an increased risk of generalized osteoporosis in adults

Common
Primary and secondary causes of gonadal insufficiency
Nutritional disorders
Thyrotoxicosis
Hyperparathyroidism
Cushing's syndrome
Insulin-dependent diabetes
Severe liver disease, especially primary biliary cirrhosis
Haemochromatosis
Osteogenesis imperfecta
Mastocytosis
Amyloidosis
Gastrectomy
Thalassaemia and chronic haemolytic disease
Malabsorption syndromes
Sarcoidosis
Adrenal atrophy and Addison's disease
Ectopic adrenocorticotrophic hormone syndrome
Tumour secretion of parathyroid hormone-related peptide
Chronic obstructive airways disease
Myelomatosis
Parenteral nutrition
Epidermolysis bullosa
Haemophilia

Uncommon in adults
Hypophosphatasia
Mastocytosis
Lymphoma and leukaemia
Congenital erythrocytic porphyria
Pregnancy

Association less certain
Acromegaly
Ankylosing spondylitis
Rheumatoid arthritis
Lactose intolerance
Endometriosis
Pernicious anaemia
Idiopathic scoliosis

MILK INTOLERANCE

Lactase deficiency may be associated with the avoidance of calcium in milk, raising the question whether this contributes to low bone mass or the risk of fracture. Population studies have given conflicting results concerning the association with osteoporosis or fracture. The most extensive study found no association of lactase deficiency with bone mass in women before or after the menopause (Slemenda *et al.*, 1991).

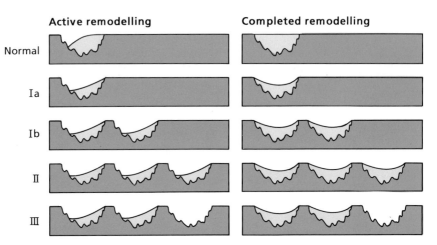

Active remodelling **Completed remodelling**

Normal

Ia

Ib

II

III

Fig. 4.4 Schematic representation of trabecular bone surfaces to illustrate the effects of myeloma on remodelling. The panels on the left depict active remodelling units and those on the right completed remodelling units. The top panels show normal bone remodelling with the infilling of a resorption bay with an equal volume of new bone (stippled) on the minority of the bone surface. The lower panels summarize histological findings in bone biopsies graded according to plasma cell burden. In stage Ia, less bone is deposited in resorption cavities than that previously resorbed so that for each remodelling sequence there is a small loss of bone. With increased plasma cell burdens (stage Ib and II), bone turnover is increased without altering this imbalance, thereby accelerating the rate of bone loss. With extensive marrow involvement (grade III) some bone resorption sites do not subsequently attract osteoblasts due to uncoupling which further accelerates bone losses. (From Taube *et al.*, 1993.)

RHEUMATOID ARTHRITIS

There is a significant association between hip fracture and rheumatoid arthritis where the risk is increased approximately twofold. The risk of vertebral fracture also appears to be increased, but this is not consistently reported.

Multifactorial cause

> This is a difficult area to study since there are many factors which complicate the disorder. These include the heterogeneity of the disease and the variable use of corticosteroids. In addition, rheumatoid arthritis itself may give rise to bone loss other than at focal sites of erosion. Patients are likely to undergo periods of local and generalized immobility, they have a decreased fat mass and these factors may contribute to bone loss.

There is some evidence that generalized bone loss may occur in patients treated only with non-steroidal anti-inflammatory agents and population-based studies suggest that the fracture risk is moderately increased (Hooyman *et al.*, 1984).

LIVER DISEASE

Chronic liver disease is commonly associated with osteoporosis, particularly primary biliary cirrhosis. It is likely that liver impairment contributes to the osteoporosis associated with alcohol abuse and haemochromatosis. In the assessment of patients with chronic liver disease, findings include a low serum phosphate (poor nutrition and decreased renal tubular reabsorption of phosphate), a low total serum calcium (due to serum albumin rather than a decrease in ionized calcium) and high serum activity of alkaline phosphatase (liver derived). These may mistakenly suggest a diagnosis of osteomalacia. Although osteomalacia may complicate chronic liver disease its frequency is low and osteoporosis is by far the more frequent finding.

Histological studies suggest that bone formation is very markedly suppressed though the number of osteoblasts is normal. This suggests that osteoblast competence is abnormal. Bone resorption as judged by urinary hydroxyproline and osteoclast counts is not abnormally increased. Increased skeletal losses may be related in part to the chronic morbidity of the associated disorders, inadequate nutrition of vitamin D, protein and possibly calcium. Severe liver disease may impair the 25-hydroxylation of vitamin D, but levels of calcidiol are not markedly reduced except in the presence of very severe disease. Other contributing factors may be the high level of endogenous circulating corticosteroids and gonadal insufficiency which may complicate chronic active hepatitis and alcoholism.

IRON RETENTION

The association of haemochromatosis with osteoporosis is well established, but it is unclear whether this is due to iron overload itself or to hypogonadism, liver disease and diabetes mellitus which complicate the disorder. Osteoporosis has been identified in 15–66% of patients with haemochromatosis and most of these have evidence of hypogonadism. Fragility fractures are also described in the absence of gonadal impairment.

The association of iron overload and osteoporosis is well documented in the Bantu of South Africa. In this tribe, haemosiderosis occurs as a result of the consumption of excessive amounts of beer containing large amounts of iron. Osteoporosis is a characteristic feature and is considered to result either from a direct toxic effect from iron overload or due to an associated deficiency of vitamin D (Lynch *et al.*, 1970). Although Bantu haemosiderosis predominantly affects middle-aged men, there are no data available on the gonadal status of affected patients. Osteoporosis has also been reported in transfusional haemosiderosis complicating thalassaemia major. Such patients were found to have low rates of bone formation and a reduced mineral apposition rate.

In chronic renal failure low rates of bone formation (aplastic bone disease) have been associated in some patients with iron rather than aluminium overload.

GASTROINTESTINAL DISEASES

Osteoporosis is associated with partial gastrectomy, inflammatory bowel disease and intestinal bypass surgery. The mechanism is not known but may be related to changes in vitamin D metabolism and the induction of mild secondary hyperparathyroidism or a functional adaptation to weight loss. Malabsorption syndromes may also give rise to osteoporosis by similar mechanisms.

CHRONIC OBSTRUCTIVE AIRWAYS DISEASE

Osteoporosis has been associated with chronic obstructive airways disease even in the absence of the use of corticosteroids. The mechanism for this is not known, but a low body mass, immobilization and smoking are likely to be contributing factors. Biochemical measurements are consistent with a reduction in the bone formation rate.

MASTOCYTOSIS

Systemic mastocytosis is a rare paraneoplastic condition characterized by diffuse multiorgan infiltration by mast cells. The organs most commonly involved include the gut, liver, spleen, lymph nodes and the skin but almost all patients have bone marrow involvement and radiographic evidence of generalized skeletal disease. Characteristically, radiographs show a stippled appearance due to a combination of sclerosis and osteopenia although one form or the other may predominate in individuals. Indeed, the disorder may occasionally present as osteoporosis where the diagnosis of mastocytosis is made on further investigation from a bone biopsy. The mechanism for

Table 4F Causes of generalized osteoporosis in children

Chromosomal disorders: Klinefelter's and Turner's syndromes, trisomy 18, trisomy 13–15
Endocrine disorders: Cushing's syndrome, thyrotoxicosis
Chronic diseases: congenital heart disease, Still's disease, chronic liver disease, coeliac disease (gluten sensitive enteropathy), cystic fibrosis
Immobilization: neuromuscular diseases and dystrophies, paralysis
Neoplasia: leukaemia
Osteogenesis imperfecta
Homocystinuria
Juvenile osteoporosis
Gaucher's disease
Hypophosphatasia
Familial dysautonomia (Riley–Day syndrome)
Lysinuric protein intolerance
Hypouricaemic and hypercalciuric osteoporosis

increased bone resorption in mastocytosis is unknown. Histologically, bone turnover in trabecular tissue is increased. Numerous mast cells are found on resorption surfaces and this is associated with an increase in osteoclast numbers. Osteoporosis is more marked at cortical than at cancellous sites and appears to respond to treatment with the bisphosphonates.

Bisphosphonates

Inherited disorders and osteoporosis in children

There are a number of disorders that may give rise to osteoporosis in children (Table 4F). A detailed consideration of their pathophysiology and features is beyond the scope of this book, but some are important to recognize since they do not invariably present in childhood but may become manifest in later life, particularly in women after the menopause. Examples include hypophosphatasia and osteogenesis imperfecta. Similarly, the presence of juvenile osteoporosis may not have been detected at the time, and only becomes evident when radiographs are taken for other reasons in adult life.

May present in adulthood

HYPOPHOSPHATASIA
Hypophosphatasia is a form of rickets or osteomalacia resulting from a generalized deficiency in bone-derived alkaline phosphatase. Serum calcium and phosphate are characteristically normal, though hypercalcaemia is an occasional association.

The age at presentation is variable. In general, the earlier the presentation the more severe the disorder (Table 4.2). Some adults are asymptomatic and others present with fragility fractures. Other adults may have generalized osteoporosis and pseudofractures which characteristically occur on the lateral aspect of the femoral cortex and differ in distribution from those associated with osteomalacia. Stress fractures occur commonly at the metatarsals and may be recurrent or heal slowly. Serum activity of alkaline phosphatase is characteristically low. The urinary excretion of phosphoethanolamine is increased and its assay is used for diagnosis. Bone biopsies show low activity of alkaline phosphatase within osteoblasts and an impaired mineralization of bone. The osteomalacia is refractory to treatment with vitamin D.

Variable presentation

OSTEOGENESIS IMPERFECTA
Osteogenesis imperfecta is an inherited disorder of connective tissue of very variable expression involving abnormalities in the synthesis or structure of type I collagen. It generally involves a single mutation in the collagen gene which renders the assembly of collagen abnormal (Byers, 1989). Many different mutations have been described and to date there is little information as to how specific mutations might account for the variable clinical expression of the disorder. The major manifestation is osteoporosis and skeletal fragility. The severity

Inherited disorder

Table 4.2 Clinical features of hypophosphatasia

Perinatal	Infantile	Childhood	Adult	Odontohypophosphatasia
Polyhydramnios	Failure to thrive	Premature loss of teeth	Premature loss of deciduous teeth	Premature loss of deciduous teeth
Stillbirth	Hypotonia	Short stature	Loss of adult teeth	No evidence of skeletal disease
Limb deformities	Rachitic deformity	Delayed walking	Osteoporosis	
Respiratory difficulties	Flail chest	Rachitic deformities	Recurrent stress fractures	
Fever	Wide fontanelles	Waddling gait	Pseudofracture	
Intracranial haemorrhage	Hypercalcaemia		Chondrocalcinosis	
Irritability	Nephrocalcinosis		Gout	
Anaemia	Craniosynostosis			
Fits	Proptosis and hyperteliorism			
	Raised intracranial pressure			

Table 4.3 Classification of osteogenesis imperfecta. (From Sillence, 1981)

Type	Inheritance	Major features
Ia	Autosomal dominant	Mild: recurrent fractures especially in childhood and in women after the menopause Blue sclerae
Ib	Autosomal dominant	As above with dentinogenesis imperfecta
II	Usually recessive	Severe: perinatal disease and lethal. Blue sclerae
III	Usually recessive	Progressive deafness Dentinogenesis imperfecta
IV	Autosomal dominant	Variable skeletal fragility White sclerae

Table 4G Features of osteogenesis imperfecta

> Osteoporosis and recurrent fractures
> Blue sclerae
> Early onset deafness
> Dentinogenesis imperfecta
> Excessive sweating
> Joint hypermobility
> Capillary fragility and thin skin
> Scoliosis
> Herniae
> High pitched voice
> Short stature
> Triangular shaped facies
> Chest deformities, triradiate pelvis and other skeletal deformities

of its clinical expression is extremely variable and the most widely used classification is that of Sillence, which provides a framework for its clinical presentation rather than for its aetiology (Table 4.3).

In childhood, osteogenesis imperfecta needs to be distinguished from Cushing's disease, juvenile osteoporosis and other rarer causes of osteoporosis (Table 4G). The differential diagnosis of multiple fractures in childhood and infancy includes child abuse. The disorder can be distinguished by its other features, particularly ligamentous laxity, joint hypermobility, fragility of the skin, dentinogenesis imperfecta and deafness. Deafness is usually conductive and less commonly sensori-neural. The sclerae may have a bluish or slate grey tint. Other associated features include a high pitched voice, short stature, scoliosis and a triangular shaped face. Deformities such as bowing may occur and this is the only form of osteoporosis where this is seen.

Blue sclerae

Patients with type I osteogenesis imperfecta commonly have a mild form of the disease with fractures in childhood. As mature adults they may have little in the way of clinical problems and present in later life with recurrent fractures, typically after the menopause (Patterson *et al.*, 1984). These patients are distinguished by their blue sclerae which, however, may fade in intensity in adult life.

There is a high frequency of deafness. A minority of patients have dentinogenesis imperfecta (type Ib). Although it is transmitted as an autosomal dominant approximately one-third of cases are new mutations, so that a family history is absent.

Radiographic findings can be very characteristic, but in adults with the mild form of the disorder they are unremarkable. In adults with little in the way of past fractures, the cortical width is normal (Patterson *et al.*, 1984). Wormian bones may be found in the sutures of the occiput but this is not a specific feature. Routine biochemical investigations are usually normal, but serum activity of alkaline phosphatase is increased following fracture.

Because of the heterogeneity of the disorder and its relative rarity, there have been no well-controlled studies examining the effects of drug intervention. Treatment, therefore, lies in the avoidance or management of fractures and maintaining maximal mobility. Experience with the use of fluoride has been disappointing, but radiographic increases in density have been observed following treatment with the bisphosphonates.

HOMOCYSTINURIA

Homocystinuria is an extremely rare inherited cause of osteoporosis, due to a deficiency in the activity of the enzyme cystathionine β-synthetase. Clinical signs first appear in childhood and include skeletal fragility, tall stature, kyphosis and/or scoliosis, genu valgum, arachnodactyly, subluxated lenses, capillary fragility and mental retardation. There are therefore similarities in the somatic expression of homocystinuria and Marfan's syndrome, but mental retardation and osteoporosis rarely occur in the latter. The cause of osteoporosis in homocystinuria is not known, but the disorder is believed to interfere with normal collagen metabolism.

JUVENILE OSTEOPOROSIS

This is a rare disorder that occurs for unknown reasons in prepubertal or adolescent children generally between the ages of 8 and 15 years. It most commonly presents with back pain due to vertebral crush fractures (Smith, 1980) which may be extensive and associated with significant loss of height. It appears to resolve spontaneously and bone loss has usually ceased by the time of presentation. Growth may be modestly impaired during the acute phase of the disorder, but catch-up growth occurs thereafter, and indeed remodelling of deformed vertebrae may occur. The fusion of ossification centres may be accelerated or delayed and the bone may be short or long and is associated with coarse trabecular marking at the epiphyses. Similar changes are observed in haemophilia. In contrast to osteogenesis imperfecta, there is no family history of fractures.

IDIOPATHIC OSTEOPOROSIS OF YOUNG ADULTS

Associations

This typically occurs between the ages of 20 and 50 years, more commonly in men than in women. It may present or be associated with hypercalciuria and nephrolithiasis. Vertebral fractures are common but it may give rise to fractures at all sites. Its cause is unknown, but a search should be made to look for known secondary causes such as alcoholism or hypogonadism. A similar syndrome occurs during or immediately after pregnancy (Smith *et al.*, 1985). The syndrome does not generally recur and counselling on this is an important part of management.

IMMOBILIZATION

Bone loss

Immobilization is an important cause of bone loss. A sedentary lifestyle has consistently been reported both in ecological and case-controlled studies to be associated with a significant increase in risk of fractures. Prospective studies show that enforced immobilization in healthy volunteers or patients results in progressive loss of bone. Progressive bone loss is a recognized complication of neurological disorders such as cerebrovascular accidents, hemiplegia and spinal cord syndromes. As much as 40% of total skeletal mass may be lost within 6 months of immobilization and give rise to fracture. Losses appear to reach a new steady state after approximately 6 months. In paraplegic patients lower limb fractures may go unrecognized. The mechanism of bone loss in terms of bone remodelling appears to be similar to that associated with gonadal insufficiency. There is an increase in the remodelling rate of bone and an imbalance between the amount resorbed and that formed (Minaire *et al.*, 1981).

The importance of weight bearing in offsetting immobilization and bone loss is suggested by the findings of progressive decreases in bone mass during space flight despite vigorous isometric exercise regimens. The nature of the signal to bone is not known but may be related to a decrease in maximum strain, a decreased number of episodes of strain or a decrease in the variety of loadings to which the skeleton is subjected.

Rapid bone loss

An elderly patient may lose the same amount of bone in 1 week of immobilization as in 1 year of the natural history of uncomplicated osteoporosis. If immobilization is transient, then bone loss is unlikely to be permanent when mobility is restored. However, prolonged immobilization or rapid losses are not associated with the restoration of the skeletal mass even if mobility is fully restored. This is discussed

Table 4H Causes of focal osteoporosis

Fractures
Immobilization
Rheumatoid arthritis
Osteomyelitis
Tuberculosis
Primary and secondary tumours
Algodystrophy
Muscular paralysis
Transient osteoporosis of the hip
Denervation or tendon rupture
Sickle cell haemoglobinopathy
Alkaptonuria

in further detail subsequently (see p. 110). An exception to this is in the young, and prolonged immobilization during childhood is more completely reversible.

Focal osteoporosis

Focal osteoporosis arises for many reasons. Those primarily related to bone disease are discussed below (Table 4H).

TRANSIENT OSTEOPOROSIS OF THE HIP
This is a rare disorder of unknown aetiology occurring most frequently in men, but also in pregnant women during the third trimester. It presents with hip pain and limitation of movement and patients may not be able to bear weight. The erythrocyte sedimentation rate may be raised. Radiographs show osteoporosis of the periarticular bone, particularly the femoral head. Symptoms generally resolve.

Regional migratory osteoporosis is also a self-limiting focal disorder of bone loss, presenting with pain usually in the lower extremities.

Table 4.4 Frequency of signs of algodystrophy in 274 patients assessed 4 weeks after Colles' fracture. (From Bickerstaff, 1990)

	Number (%)
Pain alone	0
Bone tenderness alone	1 (0.3)
Stiffness of the hand alone	7 (2.6)
Vasomotor instability alone	10 (3.6)
Two features	16 (5.8)
Three features	7 (2.6)
All four features	77 (28.1)

Note that the features most commonly coexist indicating that the components form a syndrome.

The natural history is marked by recurrences at other sites and may be similar or identical to algodystrophy.

ALGODYSTROPHY

Algodystrophy or reflex sympathetic dystrophy is a clinical syndrome characterized by pain, tenderness, dystrophic skin changes, swelling, stiffness and vascular instability (Table 4.4).

Pain at adjacent sites

The incidence of algodystrophy has been well characterized following Colles' fracture. Twenty-five to thirty percent of patients complain of pain and tenderness not at the site of the fracture but at adjacent sites, before or at the time of plaster removal. In the case of Colles' fracture tenderness is often found in the hand. It can be elicited by pressure over the bones and indeed quantifiable by dolorimetry. During the early phase of the disorder there may be swelling of the hand, but if the disorder persists swelling decreases and indeed hand volume diminishes due to atrophy of the soft tissues. A marked characteristic of algodystrophy is vasomotor and sudomotor instability. The affected part may feel warm, be discoloured and react abnormally to changes in external temperature becoming reddened or blue. Stiffness is a prominent feature.

There is gradual resolution of many of these features and in the majority of patients the disorder is self-limiting. The resolution of tenderness and vascular instability is slower than that of pain and stiffness, and appears to persist in the majority of patients for more than 1 year and in some leads to a long-term loss of function.

Trauma, the most common cause

Although 60% or more cases are associated with trauma a wide variety of other disorders has been thought to predispose to or initiate algodystrophy. In many cases, the association may be fortuitous but myocardial infarction is a common cause occurring in 10–20% of patients. Others have found a comparable incidence following cerebrovascular accidents. In 20% of cases no obvious factor is found (Doury et al., 1981).

Features

The features of swelling and bony tenderness and vascular instability of the overlying skin are less prominent at sites such as the spine or the hip. However, the other features of the disorder at these sites are sufficiently characteristic to believe that they comprise a single entity.

Radiographic changes may occur very rapidly. These comprise a generalized loss of bone density, patchy radiotranslucencies, subchondral radiotranslucencies and a loss of trabecular definition (see Chapter 5). These changes may be observed within weeks of the onset of the disorder and are associated with an increase in scintigraphic uptake on bone scans. They are, however, not specific for algodystrophy and similar to those which follow fracture or immobilization, but the changes are more marked as is the degree of bone loss. Decreases in bone density are due to an increase in cortical porosity and to a decrease in the cortical width. These are very similar again to those induced by immobilization, but the

Decreased bone density

degree of loss is significantly greater. The recovery of bone loss in uncomplicated Colles' fracture at the hand is complete within 6 months, but in the case of algodystrophy decreases in BMD have been observed for up to 1 year (Bickerstaff *et al.*, 1991). The residual deficit in cortical bone density is greater than 10% and that of the cancellous bone greater than 25%. The loss of cancellous bone is due both to a decrease in trabecular width and the disappearance of trabeculae. Partial recovery of BMD is probably achieved by hypertrophy of the remaining trabeculae and accounts for the persistence of abnormal trabecular architecture on X-rays.

FRACTURE-INDUCED OSTEOPOROSIS

Bone mass

Many investigators have reported significant reductions in bone mass after fractures of long bones, not only at the site of fractures but at adjacent sites. Losses of up to 50% have been described both proximal and distal to the fracture site. There are several reports of partial recovery of bone mass several years after fracture of the tibia but Westlin (1974) showed no restoration of lost bone 12 months after fracture of the forearm. In the lower limbs, large and sustained losses of the tibia and femur occur following leg-lengthening procedures or

Reversible in childhood

following fracture. A substantial deficit in bone mass (30%) distal to the fracture site is observed 6–9 years after fracture. Whereas irreversible deficits occur following fractures in adulthood, significant deficits are not observed in children sustaining a fracture before the age of 13 years (Fig. 4.5).

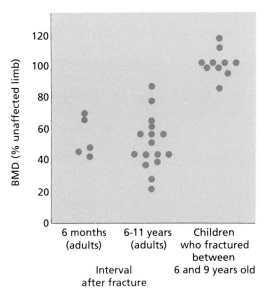

Fig. 4.5 Bone mineral density (BMD) (dual energy X-ray absorptiometry) of the distal tibia in patients following a mid-shaft fracture expressed as a percent of the contralateral site. At 6 months following fracture BMD is markedly reduced. In adults, deficits in bone density remain 6–11 years after fracture, whereas recovery is complete in children who fractured between the ages of 6 and 9 years. (From Eyres & Kanis, 1994.)

Disorders protecting against osteoporosis

Osteoarthrosis

There are very few disorders that are associated with a decreased risk of osteoporotic fracture, but osteoarthrosis may be one. It has long been noted that patients with severe osteoarthrosis of the hip may be protected from femoral neck fractures (Dequeker *et al.*, 1993), particularly intracapsular fractures. The disposition of trabecular bone is markedly altered. This may not be due solely to the focal sclerosis of bone since iliac crest biopsies from patients with osteoarthrosis at the hands have a higher cancellous bone volume than age- and sex-matched controls, a finding not confirmed for osteoarthrosis of the hip. Osteoarthrosis of the spine may also protect against vertebral fractures. Patients with osteoarthrosis are also heavier, which may contribute to increased skeletal mass but is not invariably found (Dequeker *et al.*, 1993). Another finding of possible relevance is higher growth hormone levels.

Insulin-independent diabetes

BMD in women with insulin-independent diabetes does not appear to be decreased. Indeed, bone mass is higher than normal and is related to the increase in body mass associated with type II diabetes. Some studies suggest that bone mass is increased over and above that which can be accounted for by obesity (Weinstock *et al.*, 1989), perhaps due to higher postmenopausal levels of oestrone or amylin.

References

Bickerstaff DR (1990) The natural history of post-traumatic algodystrophy. MD thesis, University of Sheffield.

Bickerstaff DR, O'Doherty DP, Kanis JA (1991) Radiographic changes in algodystrophy of the hand. *J Hand Surg*; **16B**: 47–52.

Bressot C, Meunier PJ, Chapuy MC, LeJeune E, Edouard C, Darby AJ (1979) Histomorphometric profile, pathophysiology and reversibility of corticosteroid-induced osteoporosis. *Metab Bone Dis Relat Res*; **1**: 303–311.

Byers PH (1989) Disorders of collagen biosynthesis and structure. In Scriver CR, Beaudet AL, Sly WS, Valle D (eds). *The Metabolic Basis of Inherited Disease*, 6th edn, pp. 2805–2842. McGraw-Hill, New York.

Cann CE, Henzl MR, Burrk K *et al.* (1987) Reversible bone loss is produced by the GnRH agonist nafarelin. In Cohn DV, Martin TJ, Meunier PJ (eds). *Calcium Regulation and Bone Metabolism: Basic and Clinical Aspects*, pp. 123–127. Elsevier, Amsterdam.

Christiansen P, Steiniche T, Mosekilde L, Hessor I, Melsen F (1990) Primary hyperparathyroidism: changes in trabecular bone remodelling following surgical treatment evaluated by histomorphometric methods. *Bone*; **11**: 75–79.

Delmas PD, Charhon S, Chapuy MC *et al.* (1982) Long-term effects of dichloromethylene diphosphonate (Cl$_2$MDP) on skeletal lesions in multiple myeloma. *Metab Bone Dis Rel Res*; **4**: 163–168.

Delmi M, Rapin C-H, Bengoa J-M; Delmas PD, Vasey H, Bonjour J-P (1990) Dietary supplementation in elderly patients with fractured neck of the femur. *Lancet*; **335**: 1013–1016.

Dequeker J, Johnell O, and the MEDOS study group (1993) Osteoarthritis protects against femoral neck fracture: the MEDOS experience. *Bone*; **14** (suppl 1): 51–56.

Diamond T, Stiel G, Posen S (1989) Osteoporosis in haemochromatosis: iron excess gonadal deficiency or other factors? *Ann Intern Med*; **110**: 430–436.

Doury P, Dirheimer Y, Pattin S (1981) *Algodystrophy: Diagnosis and Therapy of a Frequent Disease of the Locomotor Apparatus.* Springer-Verlag, Berlin.

Eyres KS, Kanis JA (1994) Evaluation of bone losses after tibial fractures using dual energy X-ray absorptiometry. *J Bone Joint Surg*; B: in press.

Francis RM, Peacock M, Aaron JE *et al.* (1986) Osteoporosis in hypogonadal men: role of decreased plasma 1,25-dihydroxyvitamin D, calcium malabsorption and low bone formation. *Bone*; **7**: 261–268.

Gennari C, Civitelli R (1986) Glucocorticoid-induced osteoporosis. *Clin Rheumatol*; **12**: 637–654.

Gotfredsen A, Christiansen C, Palshop T (1984) The effect of tamoxifen on bone mineral content in premenopausal women in breast cancer. *Cancer*; **53**: 853–857.

Goulding A (1981) Fasting urinary sodium/creatinine in relation to calcium/creatinine and hydroxyproline/creatinine in a general population of women. *N Z Med J*; **93**: 294–297.

Hamdy NAT, Gray RES, McCloskey EV *et al.* (1987) Clodronate in the medical management of hyperparathyroidism. *Bone*; **8**: S69–S77.

Heaney RP, Recker RR (1982) Effects of nitrogen phosphorus and caffeine on calcium balance in women. *J Lab Clin Med*; **99**: 46–55.

Heath H, Melton LJ, Chu C-P (1980) Diabetes mellitus and risk of skeletal fracture. *N Engl J Med*; **303**: 567–570.

Hordon LD, Peacock M (1990) Osteomalacia and osteoporosis in femoral neck fracture. *Bone Miner*; **11**: 147–159.

Jensen J, Nielsen LH, Lyhne N, Hallas J, Brosen K, Gram LF (1991) Drugs and femoral neck fracture: a case-controlled study. *J Intern Med*; **229**: 29–33.

Kochersberger G, Backley NJ, Leight GS *et al.* (1987) What is the clinical significance of bone loss in primary hyperparathyroidism. *Arch Intern Med*; **147**: 1951–1953.

Kyle RA (1975) Multiple myeloma: review of 869 cases. *Mayo Clin Proc*; **50**: 29–40.

Lips P, Netelenbos JC, Jongen MJM *et al.* (1982) Histomorphometric profile and vitamin D status in patients with femoral neck fracture. *Metab Bone Dis Rel Res*; **4**: 89–93.

Lynch SR, Seftel HC, Wapnick AA, Charlton RW, Bothwell TH (1970) Some aspects of calcium metabolism in normal and osteoporotic Bantu subjects with special reference to the effects of iron overload and ascorbic acid depletion. *S Afr J Med Sci*; **35**: 45–56.

Minaire P, Berard E, Meunier PJ, Edouard C, Goedert G, Pilonchery G (1981) Effects of disodium dichloromethylene diphosphonate on bone loss in paraplegic patients. *J Clin Invest*; **68**: 1086–1092.

Nordin BEC, Morris HA (1989) The calcium deficiency model for osteoporosis. *Nutr Rev*; **47**: 65–72.

Ohta H, Masuzawa T, Ikeda T, Suda Y, Makita K, Nozawa S (1992) Which is more osteoporosis-inducing, menopause or oophorectomy? *Bone Miner*; **19**: 273–285.

Patterson CR, McAllison S, Stellman JL (1984) Osteogenesis imperfecta after the menopause. *N Engl J Med*; **310**: 1694–1696.

Reid IR (1989) Pathogenesis and treatment of steroid osteoporosis. *Clin Endocrinol*; **30**: 83–103.

Ribot C, Tremollieres F, Pouilles JM, Louvet JP (1990) Bone mineral density and thyroid hormone therapy. *Clin Endocrinol*; **33**: 143–153.

Sambrook P, Birmingham J, Kempler S *et al.* (1990) Corticosteroid effects on proximal femur bone loss. *J Bone Miner Res*; **5**: 1211–1216.

Selby PL, Peacock M (1986) Ethinyloestradiol and norethisterone in the treatment of primary hyperparathyroidism in postmenopausal women. *N Engl J Med*; **314**: 1481–1485.

Sillence D (1981) Osteogenesis imperfecta: an expanding panorama of variants. *Clin Orthop*; **159**: 11–25.

Slemenda CW, Christian JC, Hui S, Fitzgerald J, Johnston CC (1991) No evidence for an effect of lactase deficiency on bone mass in pre- or postmenopausal women. *J Bone Miner Res*; **6**: 1367–1371.

Smith R (1980) Idiopathic osteoporosis in the young. *J Bone Joint Surg*; **62B**: 417–427.

Smith R, Stevenson JC, Winearis CG *et al.* (1985) Osteoporosis in pregnancy. *Lancet*; **i**: 1178–1180.

Taube T, Beneton M, McCloskey EV, Rogers S, Greaves M, Kanis JA (1993) Abnormal bone remodelling in patients with myelomatosis and normal biochemical indices of bone resorption. *Eur J Haematol*; **49**: 192–198.

Thomsen K, Gotfredsen A, Christiansen C (1986) Is postmenopausal bone loss an age-related phenomenon. *Calcif Tissue Int*; **39**: 123–127.

Weinstock RS, Goland RS, Shane E, Clemens TL, Lindsay R, Bilezikian JP (1989) Bone mineral density in women with type II diabetes mellitus. *J Bone Miner Res*; **4**: 97–101.

Westlin NE (1974) Loss of bone after Colles' fracture. *Clin Orthop*; **20**: 194–199.

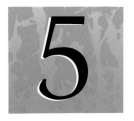

Assessment of bone mass and osteoporosis

History

As in the diagnosis and assessment of most disorders, history and physical examination are important features. In addition, there are many biochemical indices which can be measured which are either the cause of skeletal disease (e.g., increased parathyroid hormone (PTH) levels in hyperparathyroidism) or the result of changes in skeletal metabolism (e.g., increased hydroxyproline excretion in the same disorder). In addition, there are a number of radiographic features and measurements which can be used to assess osteoporosis. Bone biopsies are occasionally necessary, most notably in the assessment of osteomalacia and of renal bone disease. The use of bone density measurements is of central importance for diagnosis, prognosis and the assessment of treatment of patients with osteoporosis. These techniques and their application are reviewed briefly below.

Pivotal role of bone density

Techniques for measuring bone mass or density

A large number of techniques have been used to assess bone mass. They variously assess mineral content of the whole skeleton or particular appendicular and axial sites. The rationale for their use is dependent on the well-established relationship between the bone mineral density (BMD) and its ability to withstand compressive, tortional and bending forces. In excised bone, the correlation between the load necessary to induce skeletal failure and bone density is very high. Seventy to eighty percent of the variability in bone strength *in vitro* is determined by its mass or apparent density (Dalen *et al.*, 1976).

Rationale

> The compressive strength in cancellous bone is proportional to the square of the apparent density, so that comparatively small changes in mineral density are associated with large changes in strength.

CONVENTIONAL SKELETAL RADIOGRAPHY
Conventional radiography is relatively insensitive since bone loss is only apparent when mass has decreased by about 30–50%. There

are, however, distinctive radiographic features and morphometric techniques which may aid in the assessment of patients reviewed later in this chapter.

Sites for photodensitometry

Photodensitometric techniques have been used on X-rays to measure the optical density of the bones. The sites most commonly used have been the metacarpal and the distal radius. A reference step wedge is used alongside the area of interest and the results are usually expressed as an equivalent thickness of the wedge material. It has a reasonable

Accuracy

accuracy and there is a close correlation between measured values and bone ash, but this technique is not widely used. Computer-assisted techniques are now available and are likely to increase its value (Cosman *et al.*, 1991).

Radiogrammetry

Radiogrammetry has been used for many years to measure cortical width and is simple and inexpensive to perform. Measurements are made on X-ray films of cortical bone taken under standardized conditions. Sites assessed include the radius, humerus, femur, clavicle and tibia, but the site most commonly used is the mid-shaft of the second metacarpal. The width of bone and the cortical width of bone is measured at the midpoint of its long axis, and from this the cortical area can be derived. The mineral density of tubular bones is largely due to the cortical component and for this reason the technique has a relatively high accuracy in predicting ash weight. In the presence of marked bone loss it is less sensitive and specific, probably because it takes no account of cancellous bone density or cortical porosity.

At the metacarpal, significant bone loss has occurred when the medullary cavity diameter is equal to or greater than the combined cortical width. On the (incorrect) assumption that the metacarpals are tubular, the cortical area can be calculated and is the measurement which correlates most closely with estimates of ash weight of the metacarpals (Exton-Smith *et al.*, 1969).

SINGLE PHOTON ABSORPTIOMETRY (SPA)

SPA is widely used in the assessment of osteoporosis. It most commonly utilizes ^{125}I (27 keV) coupled with a scintillation detector which together scan across an area of interest. A disadvantage of ^{125}I is the relatively short half-life of the source (60 days). The technique

Sites for SPA

has been used at the femur, humerus, metacarpal, os calcis, hand and foot, but the most commonly used site is the forearm at the mid-radius, distal or ultradistal sites. The more distal the site the greater the contribution of cancellous bone (Table 5.1).

The amount of bone mineral in the tissue traversed by the collimated beam is derived from its attenuation through bone plus soft tissue compared to the attenuation through soft tissue alone (Mazess & Wahner, 1988). The overall thickness of the 'soft tissue' is standardized, usually by immersing the limb in water or cuffing with a fluid-filled bag. The value obtained is proportional to the bone mineral content (BMC) of the segment scanned. The value may be divided by

Table 5.1 Approximate relative contributions of cortical and cancellous bone to bone mineral measurements according to site and technique

Site	Techniques	Cortical/cancellous bone ratio
Metacarpal	SPA	98 : 2
Mid radius	SPA	95 : 5
Distal radius	SPA	80 : 20
Whole body	DXA	75 : 25
Ultradistal radius	DXA	60 : 40
Proximal femur	DXA	60 : 40
Lumbar spine (PA)	DXA	50 : 50
Trochanter	DXA	50 : 50
Os calcis	SPA	15 : 85
Lumbar spine (lateral)	DXA	10 : 90
Lumbar spine	QCT	0 : 100
Distal radius	pQCT	0 : 100

SPA, single photon absorptiometry; DXA, dual energy X-ray absorptiometry; PA, postero-anterior; QCT, quantitative computerized tomography; pQCT, peripheral QCT.

the bone width (g/cm), the area scanned (g/cm^2) or an estimate of the cross-sectional area (g/cm^2). All these measurements are often referred to as BMD. The result can be compared to that expected for gender and age (Fig. 5.1).

Errors

Because the bones of the forearm are not regular in shape and the composition of cortical and cancellous bone also varies, errors of reproducibility may be caused by variable repositioning. Problems of repositioning are less when the mid-shaft is scanned since this is

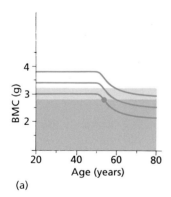

(a)

	Radius	Ulna	Total
Area scanned (cm^2)	4.22	2.53	6.75
BMD (g/cm^2)	0.432	0.357	0.404
BMC (g)	1.824	0.905	2.729
Percent of age-matched women			87.5
Percent of premenopausal women			80.5

(b)

Fig. 5.1 (a) Distal forearm scan in a 53-year-old woman. The lines give the reference range for bone mineral content (BMC) in women. The measurement, shown as a dot, lies at the lower end of the reference range for age and below the reference range for premenopausal women. The calculations are shown in (b). BMD, bone mineral density.

largely cortical bone and its mineral content does not change markedly with position. For this reason the distal and ultradistal measuring site is usually standardized by automatic site selection based on the separation of the radius and ulna.

Accuracy

The accuracy (the ability to measure what is intended) is affected by the presence of fat which has attenuation characteristics that differ from water or lean soft tissue. With some equipment, the programme assumes the fat to be a uniform shell around the bone and makes a correction, but the correction makes a number of assumptions which affect the accuracy of the method. The heterogeneity of surrounding tissues is nevertheless considerably less than those surrounding axial sites such as the spine so that estimates of accuracy are high (Nilas *et al.*, 1987). Single energy X-ray absorptiometry (SXA) has recently become available for scanning appendicular sites; the equipment uses an X-ray source and avoids, therefore, the need for isotopes.

DUAL ENERGY ABSORPTIOMETRY

Sites for dual energy absorptiometry

Axial sites, such as the spine, and proximal appendicular sites, such as the hip, cannot readily be immersed in water. In addition, these regions, particularly the vertebral bodies, are surrounded by a widely varying amount of fat, muscle mass, gut (with or without gas) and aorta (with or without atherosclerosis). These factors limit the use of SPA and SXA to the appendicular skeleton. Dual energy absorptiometry has resolved some but not all of these problems (Table 5.2). Dual photon absorptiometry (DPA) utilizes a radionucleide source of photons, usually ^{153}Gd which emits photons at two energies (44 and

Disadvantages

100 keV). Disadvantages are the cost of the isotope and its relatively short half-life (240 days). Within the past few years sources of γ radiation have been replaced by X-ray generators (Mazess & Wahner, 1988). The two effective energies required are obtained either by K-edge filtering or by rapidly switching the generator potential. The

Advantages

advantages of dual energy X-ray absorptiometry (DXA) over DPA are a higher beam intensity, and therefore faster scan, and improved spatial resolution, with more confident identification of vertebral limits and better precision.

The principles of DPA and DXA are very similar. As is the case for SPA, the source is mechanically linked to a collimated detector. Areas of interest over the bone and background are selected by the operator, assisted by the computer, and BMC in the selected area can be assessed (Fig. 5.2). Division by the length (g/cm) or area considered (g/cm^2) provides some normalization for size and, at the spine, it reduces the variation due to difficulties in defining intervertebral spaces.

Measurements

Measurements at the lumbar spine are taken in the antero-posterior position with the legs elevated to reduce the lumbar lordosis. As in the case of the forearm scan, the results can be compared to the

Table 5.2 Advantages and disadvantages of various techniques to measure bone mineral mass

Technique	Advantages	Disadvantages	Accuracy *in vivo* (%)	Precision *in vivo* (%)
QCT	Gives values of volumetric density Discriminates completely trabecular from cortical bone High resolution Low precision error (at the radius)	Comparatively high radiation dose High cost High accuracy error (single energy) Precision errors (spine)	5–10 (3–6 for forearm)	2–4 (4–6 for dual energy)
DXA	No isotopes High precision Low radiation dose Multiple sites of assessment including spine and hip	Uncertain accuracy errors *in vivo* Intermediate cost Influenced by osteoarthrosis and aortic calcification at lumbar sites	5–10 (1–2 for whole body)	1–2 (3 for lateral spine)
SPA, SXA	Low radiation High accuracy High reproducibility Low cost Portability	Restricted to appendicular sites Isotope half-life short (but not with SXA)	2–5	1–2

DXA, dual energy X-ray absorptiometry; QCT, quantitative computerized tomography; SPA, single photon absorptiometry; SXA, single energy X-ray absorptiometry.

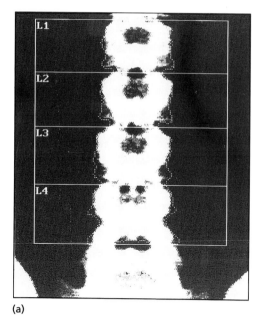

(a)

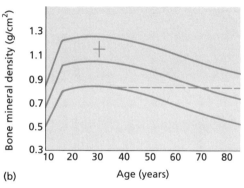

(b)

Fig. 5.2 (a) Dual energy X-ray absorptiometry scan of the lumbar spine of a healthy premenopausal woman aged 30 years. The computer has selected the edge of the spine and the vertebrae separated by the operator to give the areas of interest to be computed. (b) Plots the average bone density against the reference range for women.

young healthy reference range or that for age (Table 5.3). Although it is the vertebral body that fractures, the measurements capture not only the vertebral body, but also the arches and spinous processes which include a substantial amount of compact bone (see Table 5.1).

The presence of aortic calcification increases the apparent density and is a problem, particularly in the elderly. Radio-opaque contrast media, metallic objects, a vertebral fracture or osteoarthrosis at the

Errors

Table 5.3 Measurements made from antero-posterior scan using dual energy X-ray absorptiometry at the lumbar spine in a 53-year-old perimenopausal woman. Note the increase in vertebral area, mineral content and density with the more caudal direction. The results are compared either to the premenopausal reference range (T-score) or for an age-matched population (Z-score). In this instance the bone mineral density is 6% below the average for peak bone density but 5% above average for age

Region	Area (cm²)	Mineral content (g)	Mineral density (g/cm²)	T-score SD*	T-score (%)	Z-score SD*	Z-score (%)
L1	12.24	10.29	0.841	−0.77	91	+0.07	101
L2	13.03	13.04	1.000	−0.25	97	+0.68	108
L3	14.51	15.00	1.034	−0.46	95	+0.53	106
L4	15.08	15.81	1.048	−0.62	94	+0.39	104
Total	54.86	54.14	0.987	−0.55	94	+0.41	105

* SD units.

lumbar spine also affect the results. Vertebral fractures are usually more dense than adjacent vertebrae and can often be detected by the decrease in vertebral height or by the heterogeneity of density measured in adjacent vertebrae. In some instances radiography of the spine is required to exclude fracture, vascular calcification or arthrosis.

Lateral scanning

In order to overcome some of these problems of accuracy, a recent development has been to scan the lumbar spine in the lateral position. This has advantages in that it eliminates the posterior arch and the spines of the vertebrae as well as aortic calcification. An area within the vertebral body can also be selected. Lateral scans show greater differences in mineral density between patients with osteoporotic fractures and normal subjects than with the antero-posterior scan. Its drawbacks include the increased soft tissue mass which decreases its accuracy, and the more limited access to the lumbar vertebrae due to the ribs and pelvis which overlap the projected image.

The proximal femur is another commonly measured site and can give values for the femoral neck, trochanter, the intertrochanteric region and Ward's triangle. The whole region of the proximal femur is scanned and the sites selected with computer assistance. DPA or DXA can also be used to measure total body mineral.

QUANTITATIVE COMPUTED TOMOGRAPHY (QCT)

In QCT a thin transverse slice through the body is imaged. Under appropriate conditions the image can be quantitated to give a measure of volumetric BMD (g/cm^3 or g/ml) and cancellous bone can be measured independently of surrounding cortical bone and aortic calcification.

Costs

Capital and running costs of X-ray QCT systems are so high that an installation solely for bone mineral measurement is not generally feasible. Nevertheless, the possibility of measuring cancellous bone in the vertebrae rather than the integral of compact and cancellous bone (as with DXA and DPA) has attracted considerable attention (Cann, 1988). A dedicated forearm scanner has also been developed which uses ^{125}I as a photon source. The precision errors *in vivo* are relatively low (2–5%). The biggest source of error in single energy X-ray QCT systems is due to fat within the bone marrow. Large accuracy errors (up to 30%) may occur (Mazess, 1983) but can be markedly decreased by carrying out scans at two different potentials. The radiation dose of QCT is significantly higher than with absorptiometric techniques.

Forearm scanner

Errors

ULTRASOUND EVALUATION OF BONE

Several methods have been developed which variously examine the velocity, attenuation or reflection of ultrasound. The interest in their use is that they do not involve ionizing radiation and may give some information concerning the structural organization of bone in addition to bone mass or density. In addition, the equipment is generally portable.

Ultrasound attenuation

This method has not yet been extensively validated, but the results are sufficiently encouraging to warrant consideration in the future outside the realms of clinical research (Langton *et al.*, 1984; Palmer & Langton, 1987). So far only the os calcis has been examined. The system consists of a water tank containing two broadband ultrasonic transducers, one acting as a transmitter, the other as a receiver, at a fixed separation, together with a computer-interfaced electronic generation and detection unit. A short burst of ultrasound is passed through the heel, the frequency varying from 200 to 1000 kHz. The attenuation at each frequency is compared with that from water alone. The slope of the linear portion of this difference plotted against frequency is measured. The attenuation is related to both the amount of bone in the path of the ultrasound and to the trabecular structure. The reproducibility in patients ranges from 2.5 to 3.5% (McCloskey *et al.*, 1990).

Trabecular structure

Ultrasound velocity and reflection

Ultrasound reflection may also provide some index of the material properties of bone, but has not been widely studied. Several techniques have been developed to measure the velocity of ultrasound in bone. The speed of sound is proportional to the square root of the product of the stiffness or modulus of elasticity and the bone density. It is not yet known whether the speed of sound provides a measure of bone 'quality' and provides an assessment of bone fragility over and above that captured by absorptiometric measurements alone.

Quality of bone

OTHER TECHNIQUES

Several other techniques to measure bone mineral have been developed but their current use is largely confined to clinical research. These include photon scattering methods which allow the possibility of measuring cancellous bone without interference from the surrounding cortex.

Neutron activation analysis

Neutron activation analysis (NAA) has been widely used to measure bone mineral. When the area to be examined is irradiated with neutrons, a proportion of ^{48}Ca is converted to ^{49}Ca and can be quantified by examining the characteristic γ-ray emission. The half-life of ^{49}Ca is only 8.8 minutes. NAA has been used to measure bone mineral at many sites but the development of DXA has made many of its skeletal applications redundant.

Comparison of techniques

The performance characteristics of the most widely used techniques are listed in Table 5.2. With the exception of QCT, the doses of radiation with all these techniques are low. A useful way of comparing them is against the natural background radiation incurred each year (100%). In this context, the dose received by an AP scan of the lumbar spine is 0.03% of the background dose. Higher doses occur with lateral scanning (0.1%) and even with QCT it is only 2% of the yearly background radiation, equivalent to the additional radiation incurred from a transatlantic flight (1.7%).

Diagnosis of osteoporosis

Diagnosis in women

The use of these techniques for the diagnosis of osteoporosis in women is relatively straightforward. A BMC or BMD value at or below 2.5 SD of the mean in young adult women is appropriate for the diagnosis of osteoporosis (see Chapter 1), but different criteria should be used in men and in children.

Difficulties

Bone mineral mass measurements have several general limitations as well as limitations specific to a particular methodology, which are important for the investigator or physician to recognize. The test may become difficult to interpret in the presence of other disorders, particularly in the presence of osteomalacia. A low BMC can only be interpreted as measuring a low bone mass where the bone tissue itself is normally mineralized. Osteoarthrosis, vascular calcification, fracture and scoliosis also impair interpretation depending on the site chosen. The test is influenced by overlying metal objects and by contrast media. In addition, none of the techniques, with the exception of QCT, give measurements of true BMD. For example, SXA, SPA and DXA provide information on BMC (g) which can be adjusted, for example, to the area of the vertebral bodies visualized to give an estimate of apparent areal density (BMD; g/cm^2). Other adjustments include muscle mass and the width of bone. It is important to recognize that each adjustment incurs errors. For example, at the spine, adjustment for area overestimates density in large individuals and underestimates this in those with small bones. Despite these caveats, any of these techniques may be reliably used to diagnose osteoporosis.

COMPARISON OF SITES

Despite the large differences in skeletal composition between sites (see Table 5.1), highly significant correlations between sites are reported in the case of healthy populations. The correlation between sites is somewhat less in the elderly. Thus, to diagnose vertebral osteoporosis, measurements at the spine are appropriate whereas other sites are more appropriate in other circumstances. Within the limitations of accuracy (discussed on p. 121), a diagnosis of generalized osteoporosis can be made from any site. Given the choice of a site, measurements made by different techniques give similar results. For example, both SPA and DXA perform similarly *in vivo* in assessing the calcium content at the forearm. There are close correlations

Vertebral osteoporosis

in the order of 0.8–0.9 between vertebral densities assessed by QCT, DXA or DPA and even higher comparing DXA and QCT *ex vivo*.

COMPARATIVE ACCURACY

All techniques incur some error of accuracy. Systematic inaccuracies occur particularly at the spine since the vertebrae are irregular in shape and apparent density and mineral content will depend in part upon the algorithm utilized for edge detection. It is important therefore that values are interpreted alongside an appropriate reference range obtained with the same equipment. Non-systematic errors of accuracy also occur which means that ash weight will be predicted less confidently from BMD. Both SPA and DXA measure BMC within a defined area and variable positioning will alter the projected areal density value obtained. At the spine, areas also include intervertebral discs which may also give rise to non-systemic errors. In addition, the presence of osteophytes and soft tissue (especially aortic) calcification will also be included and, as mentioned, may make a significant contribution to apparent BMD. Some of these factors are of less concern in younger women but the prevalence of spinal osteoarthrosis is high at the age of the menopause.

Errors caused by fat

The largest source of error in accuracy arises because of variable soft tissue density. The theory of dual energy techniques requires that there are only two components present: bone and soft tissue of uniform composition. In practice fat forms a further component with attenuation characteristics which differ from water, muscle or most organs. A uniform layer does not matter, but fat is distributed non-uniformly in the region of the lumbar spine. Errors of spine bone mineral of up to 10% can be introduced. An error can also be introduced by fat within the vertebral bone marrow. Fat content increases with age and complicates the assessment of individuals and their response to some types of treatment including oestrogens and anabolic steroids.

Comparative accuracy

The estimate of accuracy most relevant to diagnostic use in patients is that derived as closely as possible from the situation *in vivo*, such as studies from cadavers. Estimates of accuracy are given in Table 5.2. The accuracy has to be considered alongside the variance in bone mineral that occurs in the population to be examined, which ranges from 10 to 50%, depending upon the technique and any normalization procedures applied (Kanis *et al.*, 1983). For example, a technique with an accuracy error of more than 10% cannot be used to determine whether a patient has osteoporosis where the population variance is in the order of 20% or less. Of the techniques widely available, the accuracy performance in relation to the population variance is highest in the case of SPA by a factor of twofold or so (Kanis *et al.*, 1990). This might suggest that SPA should be the technique of choice for diagnosis utilizing a single estimate of bone density, but an appendicular measurement (at the wrist) is approximately twofold weaker than DXA at predicting bone mass at the spine or hip so that there is little to choose between them.

Assessment of bone loss and gain

Measurements of bone loss or bone gain have an obvious application in the study of the natural history of osteoporosis and the effects of treatment. The most direct method of assessing bone loss or gain is by repeated measurements of bone mass but several factors determine the suitability of bone mass measurements for measuring rates of bone loss with confidence. Apparent changes are open to misinterpretation, for example, if the width of the bone increases with age or if there is an age-related increase in extraskeletal calcification. Changes in the distribution of fat can lead to additional artefacts. As mentioned, the fat fraction of lumbar bone increases by about 7% per decade in both men and women, which will lead to an overestimate of bone loss. The apparent anabolic effects of oestrogens or anabolic steroids on skeletal density are partly due in part to a significant decrease in fatty tissue surrounding bone. Similarly, increases in bone density ascribed to exercise may be due in part to a decrease in body fat, an increase in lean body mass or both.

Difficulties

The probability of detecting a difference between two measurements (when a difference truly exists) depends upon the confidence that can be placed on the single (or repeated) measurement. For this reason, individuals must be followed for longer periods with less precise techniques to be sure that a given change or lack of change has really occurred (Table 5.4). The relevant estimates of precision in this context are those obtained in osteoporotic patients, where the errors are greater than in health or with phantoms (see Table 5.2). Precision errors have to be judged against the rates of bone loss expected in an individual. The average postmenopausal bone loss over 1 year is about 2%, i.e., of the same order as the precision of SPA, SXA and DXA. This might suggest that average or greater than average rates of bone loss can be detected with confidence within 2 years by a repeated measurement, but slower losses would take longer to detect.

Precision

Although the average rate of bone loss is 2% there is a three- to fivefold range in loss depending on the site (Hansen *et al.*, 1991). It is lower at cortical than at cancellous sites. Thus, the ratio of loss to precision error is more favourable for DXA than for SPA. Rates of bone loss decline several years after the menopause so that a longer interval between measurements is required to evaluate a given change. An interval of 5 years is likely to be more than adequate to assess rates of loss in the majority of osteoporotic individuals, but this interval is less than optimal for many clinical purposes such as assessing the responses to treatment. This may require yearly assessments depending on the change anticipated, the intervention used

Interval between measurements

Table 5.4 Duration of study necessary to determine significant bone loss ($P<0.05$) in an individual patient. (From Kanis *et al.*, 1983)

Rate of bone loss (% per year)	Reproducibility (CV %)	Minimum duration of study (years)
1	1	2
	2	4
	5	8
	10	16
2	1	1
	2	2
	5	4
	10	8
5	1	1
	2	1
	5	2
	10	3

CV, coefficient of variation.

and the reproducibility of the technique. For example, with the use of sodium fluoride, increases in cancellous bone mass of 5–10% may occur within 1 year of treatment. In this case a repeat assessment at 1 year would be adequate to determine whether an individual had responded to treatment.

Response to treatment

Assessment of fracture risk

Prognostic use

A third use of measurements of bone mineral is to assess the probability of future fractures. Many prospective studies show that the risk increases the lower the measurement of bone mass. The gradient of risk lies between 1.5 and 2.8 for each SD drift in BMD (Fig. 5.3). Such studies provide a basis for the assessment of sensitivity and specificity of bone mineral measurements used in this way. These should not be based, however, upon fracture risk over a finite period of observation. A woman with a low BMD who has not fractured over a 5-year interval but will do so 10 years later cannot be considered as a false-positive. In the context of a lifetime risk, rather than the presence of a fracture, true-positive rate is defined as the proportion of individuals who would in their lifetime sustain a fracture with a BMD test value below a defined cut-off range. The true-negative rate is defined as the proportion of subjects who would not fracture in their lifetime with values for BMD above the cut-off value.

Sensitivity and specificity

Table 5.5 presents estimates of 'sensitivity' and 'specificity' under a number of different conditions. The gradient of risk of future fracture for each SD shift in BMD is shown at 1.5, 2.0 or 2.5, which covers conservatively the range identified in prospective studies. The average

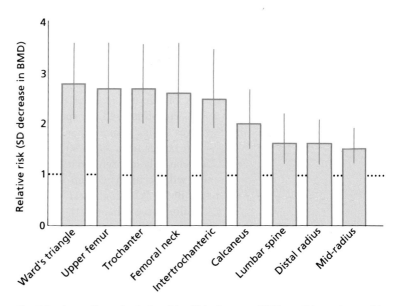

Fig. 5.3 Age-adjusted relative risk of hip fracture (95% confidence intervals) for each SD decrease in bone mineral density (BMD) at the site shown. Data based on measurements with dual energy X-ray absorptiometry in 8134 women aged 65 years or more followed for a mean of 1.8 years. (From Cummings *et al.*, 1993.)

lifetime risk of fracture is given as 15 and 30%. The former is an accurate assessment of hip fracture risk in Europe and the United States, and the latter a conservative assessment of the risk of any osteoporotic fracture (see Chapter 1). Specificity and sensitivity are

Table 5.5 Estimates of sensitivity and specificity of a single measurement of bone mass to predict hip fracture (15% lifetime risk) or osteoporotic fracture (30% risk) in postmenopausal women. Values are given where the risk of fracture is assumed to increase by 1.5, 2.0 or 2.5 for each SD decrease in bone mineral density. (From WHO, 1994)

| | | High-risk category (% population) | | | | | |
| | | 6.5 | | | 30 | | |
Gradient of risk	Lifetime risk (%)	Sensitivity (%)	Specificity (%)	Accuracy (%)	Sensitivity (%)	Specificity (%)	Accuracy (%)
1.5	15	38	98	89	65	75	74
	30	29	100	79	58	78	72
2	15	47	100	92	75	77	77
	30	31	100	79	68	80	76
2.5	15	52	100	93	81	77	78
	30	35	100	81	74	80	78

calculated assuming the high-risk category is 6.5 or 30% of the perimenopausal population (i.e., the range over which intervention might be contemplated).

When considered in this way the false-positive rate is close to zero, indicating a high specificity of bone mineral measurements since the lifetime risk of fracture is close to 100% using the 6.5% cut-off. When a 30% cut-off is used the specificity remains high (over 75%) over all ranges of risk assumptions. In contrast, the test lacks sensitivity, which ranges from 29 to 80% depending on the assumptions made. The relatively low sensitivity indicates that a large proportion of fractures will occur in women who lie in the lower risk groups when using BMD as a single test to assess fracture risk. To use a previous analogy (see Chapter 1), many patients who suffer from stroke are normotensive but most patients with severe untreated hypertension will have a stroke.

Sensitivity increases with the gradient of risk assumed. This indicates that tests with improved accuracy would increase the sensitivity of the test. Accuracy can be improved by site-specific measurements. The gradient of vertebral fracture risk for measurements made at the spine is higher than for density measurements made of the hip or forearm. Conversely, measurements made at the hip predict hip fracture more confidently than measurements made elsewhere (see Fig. 5.3).

Thus, site-specific measurements, though they do not improve the prediction for all fractures, do improve the prediction for fractures at that particular site.

INTERVENTION THRESHOLDS
Because of the continuous distribution of bone density, the relationship between fracture risk and density is stochastic. The choice of an intervention threshold is for this reason arbitrary. A reasonable cut-off in women with high specificity and adequate sensitivity is to consider the lowest quintile of BMC (the highest quintile at risk) of the healthy female population at significant future risk of fracture. In developing a management strategy, it may be of value to identify an additional group at intermediate risk (the fourth quintile of risk) in whom further assessment, such as rates of bone loss, might be justified.

This cut-off point is relevant where the aims of treatment are to decrease the risk of all osteoporotic fractures. More stringent cut-offs would be appropriate if the aim were solely to prevent hip fractures, perhaps the lowest 5% rather than the lowest quintile. Moreover, if hip fractures were the only concern, it would be more appropriate to measure risk at the hip where the gradient of risk is greater.

Because life-expectancy decreases with age, the lifetime risk of fractures of the hip and wrist are comparable at all ages after the menopause (Cummings, 1985). At all ages the risk of osteoporotic fractures increases with decreasing BMD. Indeed, the gradient of risk with BMD is if anything higher in the elderly (Hui *et al.*, 1988). Thus, choosing the lowest quintile for BMD of an appropriate age-matched population will have a similar specificity. An alternative approach is to set an intervention threshold more closely related to a given lifetime risk. Models have been created to permit the estimation of lifetime fracture risks for any given bone mass and age (Suman *et al.*, 1993). This approach could be useful to select patients for treatment whose lifetime risk was at a certain level irrespective of age.

Biochemical assessment of osteoporosis

Indirect indices of skeletal metabolism provide a valuable tool for the assessment of patients and sometimes for the evaluation of treatment. In contrast to the focal assessment of disease by bone histology, regional assessments of bone mass or radiography, biochemical indices of disease activity provide an integrated assessment of the activity of the underlying disorder. Disease activity has been assessed in terms of calcium metabolism, collagen turnover and indices of the functional activity of bone cells themselves.

Integrated assessment

SERUM AND URINE CALCIUM
In uncomplicated osteoporosis serum calcium and phosphate values are not markedly disturbed: nor are its urinary measurements, reflecting relatively slow rates of bone loss, the coupling of calcium accretion and resorption rates in bone, and the integrity of many of the normal homeostatic mechanisms. In all forms of generalized osteoporosis there is nevertheless an increased net efflux of calcium from bone. This represents a small challenge to serum calcium, but this is further offset by a decrease in intestinal absorption of calcium so that the 24-hour urinary excretion of calcium usually lies within the laboratory reference range. Hypercalciuria, if present, indicates increased intestinal absorption of calcium or markedly accelerated rates of bone resorption, much greater than that of uncomplicated osteoporosis. An exception is the hypercalciuria of immobilization which is most characteristically seen when the metabolic activity of bone is high such as in Paget's disease, hyperparathyroidism, after fracture or in the young.

Calciuria

In the postabsorptive state, the contribution of intestinal absorption to calcium excretion is minimized. Thus, measurements of calcium excretion are made from a sample of fasting urine taken in the postabsorptive state after an overnight fast which diminishes the effect of diet. Variations in the concentration of calcium are adjusted by dividing the result by the concurrent creatinine concentration. An increased fasting calcium excretion suggests increased bone resorption, suppressed formation or both. High fasting urinary excretion rates are found particularly in the initial 6–10 years after the menopause and in both sexes with secondary causes of osteoporosis. There is a large overlap between reference ranges and values found in patients with osteoporosis, so that it has little value in the diagnosis of osteoporosis (Fig. 5.4).

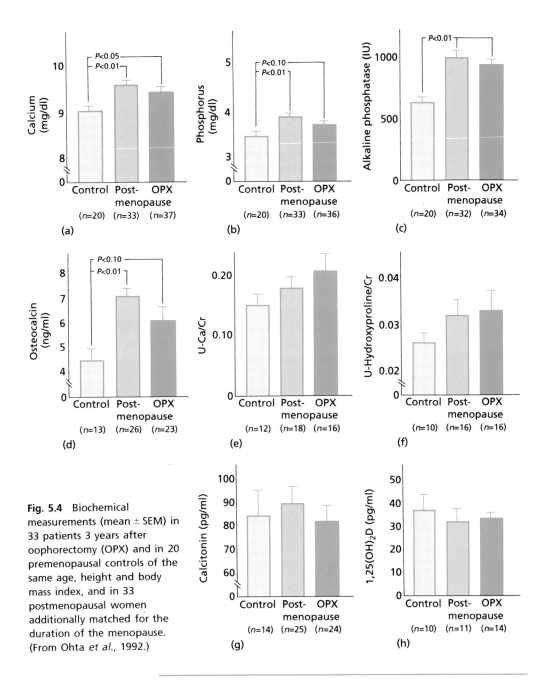

Fig. 5.4 Biochemical measurements (mean ± SEM) in 33 patients 3 years after oophorectomy (OPX) and in 20 premenopausal controls of the same age, height and body mass index, and in 33 postmenopausal women additionally matched for the duration of the menopause. (From Ohta et al., 1992.)

As would be expected, the fasting urinary excretion of calcium is decreased by treatments which decrease bone resorption, increase bone formation or both. This measurement can be used to monitor treatment with oestrogens, the bisphosphonates, calcitonin and other inhibitors of bone resorption.

Several more specific indices of skeletal metabolism have been developed. The most common are the serum activity of alkaline phosphatase, serum osteocalcin and the urinary excretion of hydroxyproline.

ALKALINE PHOSPHATASE

Activity of alkaline phosphatase is the most frequently used biochemical marker of skeletal disease. Alkaline phosphatase is derived in part from osteoblasts. In healthy individuals about half of the activity of alkaline phosphatase in serum is derived from bone and the remainder from liver. The bone and liver enzymes differ only in their post-translational modification. There may also be contributions to serum activity from the intestine and other tissues including the placenta in pregnancy. Tests which distinguish the bone-derived isoenzyme have been developed and are likely to become more widely used.

In patients with osteoporosis, the activity of alkaline phosphatase may be moderately increased for several reasons. Immediately after the menopause values of alkaline phosphatase increase approximately twofold due to the generalized increase in bone turnover (see Fig. 5.4). Similar increments in activity occur with several disorders causing osteoporosis such as hyperparathyroidism and thyrotoxicosis. Secondly, increased serum activity of alkaline phosphatase also occurs because of focal disturbances of bone metabolism, most commonly due to fractures. Values increase within a week, remain high over a period of several months and subside thereafter, which is important to recognize when screening patients for osteomalacia. Serum activity of alkaline phosphatase rarely exceeds twice the upper limit of the laboratory reference range. Changes greater than this should alert the physician to seek other causes, either due to skeletal disease, for example Paget's disease or osteomalacia, or due to non-skeletal sources of alkaline phosphatase such as the liver. Significant contributions from extraskeletal tissues can be excluded by isoenzyme studies or, more usually, by the measurement of other hepatic enzymes such as 5'-nucleotidase or γ-glutamyl transferase. Account needs to be taken of the day to day variations. Based on repeated estimates in patients with osteoporosis increases in activity of greater than 30% exceed the day to day variation expected by chance.

HYDROXYPROLINE

Urinary excretion of hydroxyproline provides the second major biochemical marker used to monitor skeletal disease. Collagen is the major protein of bone and skin, and most hydroxyproline of endogen-

Sources

Osteoporotic patients

Fracture

ous origin that is excreted in urine (perhaps 90%) comes from the turnover of collagen in these tissues. When bone turnover is increased, the relative skeletal contribution to total excretion is correspondingly increased.

A major difficulty in the use of hydroxyproline is that it is a rather laborious chemical measurement. In addition, the day to day variation is twice that of serum alkaline phosphatase. A further problem is that there is a significant dietary source from food products. It is traditional to measure hydroxyproline, therefore, after restricting the collagen and gelatin intake of patients. This makes it necessary to avoid meats, gravies, ice-creams and several other foods. This difficulty can be overcome to some extent by collecting urine after an overnight fast. The use of a fasting-spot urine also avoids the need for timed collections since the hydroxyproline concentration is expressed as a ratio to creatinine concentration. Laboratory ranges vary but in our own laboratory the upper limit of normal is less than 30 mmol/mol of creatinine. Values increase approximately twofold after the menopause (Crilly et al., 1980).

OSTEOCALCIN

Osteocalcin, also known as bone γ-carboxyglutamic acid containing protein, is the most abundant non-collagenous protein in bone and is thought to be synthesized exclusively by osteoblasts. It is also found in serum, and for these reasons there has been considerable interest in its assay as a possible means for the evaluation of patients with bone disease, particularly in osteoporosis.

Histological studies have shown significant correlations between the rates of bone formation and serum values for osteocalcin. As expected, the correlations between indices of resorption and serum osteocalcin were less marked (Brown et al., 1984). Serum values for osteocalcin have been shown to increase following immobilization and for several years after the menopause, and are a more sensitive index of the postmenopausal increase in bone turnover than either total alkaline phosphatase or urinary hydroxyproline (see Fig. 5.4). Care is required in interpreting values in the presence of renal failure since the kidney is a site of its metabolism.

OTHER BIOCHEMICAL INDICES OF SKELETAL METABOLISM

Because of the non-specificity and limitations in the routine assessment of bone turnover in osteoporosis, there has been great interest in the development of more specific indices of skeletal metabolism.

They have been extensively used to explore the dynamics of bone disease and to test therapeutic interventions and, because of their specificity and low precision errors of measurement, also have a role in the assessment of individuals. Those evaluated in osteoporosis are shown in Table 5.6. There are several assays for deoxypyridinoline

Table 5.6 Biochemical markers of disease activity used in osteoporosis. (From Kanis, 1991)

Measurement	Source	Osteoporosis
Formation		
Alkaline phosphatase	Liver/bone/gut	Increased
Skeletal alkaline phosphatase	Bone: osteoblasts	Increased
Osteocalcin	Bone: osteoblasts	Increased
Procollagen peptides	Bone: osteoblasts	Increased
Decarboxylated osteocalcin	Bone: osteoblasts	Increased
Resorption		
Tartrate-resistant acid phosphatase	? Osteoclasts	Increased
Deoxypyridinoline and pyridinolone	Collagen cross-links	Increased

which have been well validated as an index of bone resorption in the context of osteoporosis and are used routinely in some centres.

BIOCHEMICAL ESTIMATION OF BONE LOSS

Usage

A major interest in the use of biochemical indices of skeletal metabolism has been to assess disease activity and rates of bone loss. A single measurement of bone mass does not indicate whether bone is currently being lost or whether it was lost in the past. In asymptomatic individuals at risk from osteoporosis, an assessment of bone loss may aid in the decision whether to offer a therapeutic intervention, since the time to reach an osteoporotic state will depend on the rate of loss as well as on the current bone mass. The assessment of disease activity can help determine the effect of treatment and relapse. The biochemical assessment of rates of bone loss has the potential advantage of avoiding the need for repeated assessments of bone density.

Which index?

The greatest interest in this application has been to assess bone loss at the time of the menopause. At this time, the biochemical estimates of both bone resorption and formation increase markedly in the order of 30–100% (Stepan *et al.*, 1987) and also decrease after treatment with gonadal steroids. An increase in bone resorption precedes the increase in formation at the menopause so that information on both aspects of remodelling improves estimates of rate of bone loss. Those indices shown to be of value are serum activity of alkaline phosphatase and its skeletal isoenzyme, serum osteocalcin, the fasting calcium/creatinine ratio and hydroxyproline/creatinine ratios in urine. The measurement of pyridinoline cross-links provide similar information as hydroxyproline, and suitable assays have recently become available.

Prospective clinical studies suggest that rates of loss can be predicted from a panel of biochemical estimates in the early postmenopausal years. The higher the level of bone turnover, the more bone resorption increases compared with bone formation and the higher the rate of bone loss. Although bone loss is not linear, it has been shown that biochemical markers can predict the change in BMD, at least for up to 12 years after the menopause (Fig. 5.5). The degree of correlation between bone loss measured directly and that judged indirectly by biochemical tests suggests that biochemical tests have an efficiency of 50% or more compared to that of direct sequential measurements of bone mass. They are likely, therefore, to improve the stratification of fracture risk.

Radiographic assessment of osteoporosis

The diagnosis of osteoporosis can often be made from X-rays, albeit with low sensitivity. A generalized decrease in the apparent density of bone is often termed osteopenia. The major causes of osteopenia are osteoporosis, osteomalacia, hyperparathyroidism irrespective of its cause and the generalized rarefaction of bone found in some patients with neoplasia. With the exception of osteomalacia these other causes might arguably also be termed osteoporosis in the sense that mineralized bone mass is decreased. Nor too is the distinction between osteomalacia, secondary hyperparathyroidism, and osteoporosis always straightforward (see Chapters 2 and 4). Nevertheless, the finding of osteopenia on X-rays is most commonly due to osteoporosis.

The additional radiographic features of generalized osteoporosis include abnormalities in trabecular architecture, a decrease in cortical width and the fractures that arise. Evidence for pre-existing fractures

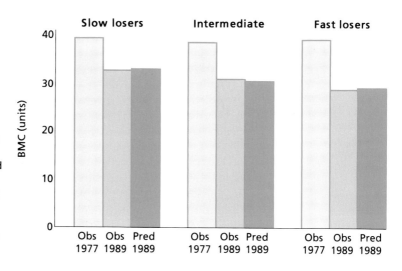

Fig. 5.5 Observed (Obs) bone mineral content (BMC) at baseline (1977) and 12 years later (1989) compared to the levels predicted (Pred) by baseline bone mass and biochemical tests for slow, intermediate and fast losers of bone in the postmenopausal period. (Modified from Hansen *et al.*, 1991.)

are prominent in the spine since the deformities induced are generally not reversible, except in young children.

Osteopenia is more marked at the spine and pelvis than the appendicular skeleton in the early stage of hypogonadal osteoporosis, presumably related to the high content of cancellous bone at these sites and the greater early rate of loss compared with cortical bone. Changes in the skull are not marked though bone loss occurs there after the menopause, but can be a marked feature of Cushing's disease, juvenile osteoporosis, hyperparathyroidism and hyperthyroidism. Sites most commonly used in the assessment of patients are the spine, hip and hands.

SPINE

There are several problems in determining a reduction in bone volume at the spine from plain radiography. Thirty percent or more of skeletal tissue must be lost before becoming readily apparent. Also, the apparent density is markedly affected by surrounding fat. In obese subjects vertebral bodies appear more osteopenic than those in their leaner counterparts. Finally, differences in technical factors such as the energy used have an important effect. Within these limitations, osteoporosis preferentially affects the central portion of the cancellous bone of the vertebral bodies, so that if the density in this region is equal to or less than that of soft tissues then this is a reliable sign of osteoporosis. In addition, the junction between the end-plate and cancellous bone becomes more distinct so that the apparent density of the end-plates becomes enhanced (Fig. 5.6).

In postmenopausal osteoporosis trabecular numbers decrease. The

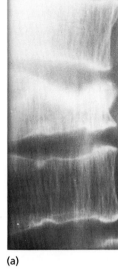 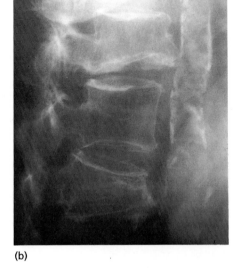

Fig. 5.6 Lateral thoracic (a) and lumbar (b) radiographs. Note the apparent accentuation of the vertebral end-plates due to osteopenia of the vertebral bodies. Note also the accentuation of vertical trabeculae in the thoracic spine.

(a) (b)

remaining trabeculae hypertrophy, particularly the vertical trabeculae. The preferential loss of horizontal trabeculae and hypertrophy of vertical bars give rise to a striated appearance (see Fig. 5.6). These changes in trabecular markings contrast with those observed in glucocorticoid-induced osteoporosis or in osteomalacia. In these disorders, trabecular markings usually become indistinct giving rise to a fuzzy or ground-glass appearance. The reason relates to the more perfectly preserved trabecular network and the lack of trabecular hypertrophy. An additional feature of corticosteroid-induced osteoporosis is the persistence of callus following fracture, which gives rise to the appearance of pseudocallus (Fig. 5.7) which can be particularly marked at vertebral sites. Pseudocallus may be found in the absence of overt vertebral deformities, and presumably reflects the exuberant callus formation that occurs with microfracture.

In children a bone-within-bone appearance may occur due to the deposition of osteoporotic bone during growth. This may be observed in many disorders but is most common in congenital heart disease. It is also found as a normal variant in infants 1 month or so after birth and resolves spontaneously.

Vertebral deformity

The characteristic deformities which occur in osteoporosis are due to central compression fractures, anterior wedge deformity and complete collapse of the vertebral bodies (see Fig. 2.1). None are specific to osteoporosis nor are vertebral deformities solely caused by osteoporosis. Even in the context of osteoporosis the term deformity rather than fracture is commonly used since the cut-off point between a normal variation and a fracture is not well defined, and a number of technical artefacts may give the appearance of deformity.

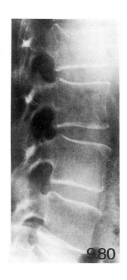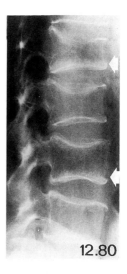

Fig. 5.7 Progression of glucocorticoid-induced osteoporosis over a 3-month interval. Note the lack of trabecular markings in contrast to postmenopausal osteoporosis (see Fig. 5.6). Over this period, osteopenia became more marked so that apparent density at the vertebral body is less than that of the disc space. In addition, pseudocallus has arisen in association with vertebral deformities. (Courtesy of Professor R. Maldague.)

An oblique projection may give the appearance of a central compression fracture. For this reason radiographs should be adequately centred. For quantitative vertebral morphometry two lateral radiographs of the spine are taken centred on T7 and L2. The taking of films during inspiration blurs the ribs and improves the definition of vertebral geometry. In assessing vertebral shape in this way, account needs to be made for the normal variations that occur within the spine and between spines. The posterior height is usually several millimetres greater than the anterior height, except in the lower lumbar region where the converse holds true. The absolute height measured will depend on the magnification of the vertebral bodies. For this reason most investigators utilize ratios, for example the anterior/posterior height ratio. Normal ranges (for ratios) are similar in white people in Europe and North America but differ in other races.

A variety of criteria have been developed to distinguish normal from abnormal vertebrae (McCloskey *et al.*, 1993). The incidence and prevalence of vertebral osteoporosis depends critically on the criteria chosen (see Chapter 1), but does not affect the general description of the types of vertebral fracture.

A wedge fracture describes a vertebra with a reduced anterior height but normal posterior height. Biconcave or central fractures describe a decrease in central height compared to the anterior and posterior borders. A compression fracture is a reduction in all three heights. Posterior wedging other than of L4 or L5 is not a feature of osteoporosis and is usually an unstable fracture due to trauma, neoplasia or other causes.

The biconcavity of vertebral bodies following central compression fracture gives rise to the term cod-fish vertebrae since they resemble the vertebral bodies of fish. Biconcavity may be associated with discal herniations or 'Schmorl's nodes', which arise because of pressure from adjacent vertebral discs on the thinned cortex. Schmorl's nodes are not specific for osteoporosis and occur in any disorder where there is incompetence of the end-plate. Indeed, in some series they are so common that their causal association with osteoporosis has been questioned.

Central compression fractures are particularly common in the mid-thoracic spine whereas anterior-wedge fractures are more common in the lower thoracic region. Fractures occurring above T5 are sufficiently unusual in osteoporosis that other pathology should be suspected.

There are some normal variants in vertebral shape which should not be confused with end-plate deformities. Central compressions should be distinguished from the concavity which occurs as a normal variant of the lower surface of lumbar vertebrae. A wide variety of other disorders gives rise to changes in vertebral shape. Scheuermann's disease is osteochondrosis of the secondary ossification centres of the vertebral bodies. It commonly occurs between the ages of 12 and 16 years and may give rise to back pain, a dorsal kyphosis and deformities of the vertebral bodies (Fig. 5.8). The vertebral bodies appear wedge shaped and the intervertebral disc spaces may be narrowed with calcification. There may also be central compressions, but unlike those in osteoporosis there are surface irregularities. The margins of the vertebral bodies are absent, either because of defective

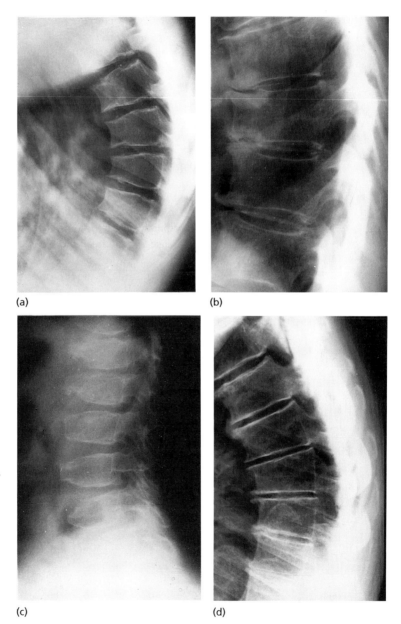

(a) (b)

(c) (d)

Fig. 5.8 (a) and (b) Anterior deformities due to Scheuermann's disease. Note the kyphosis due to anterior wedging of the vertebral bodies (a). The end-plates are irregularly shaped in contrast to anterior crush fracture (b). (c) Shows spondylo-epiphyseal dysplasia of the lumbar spine and (d) generalized osteoarthrosis (courtesy J. Dequeker).

formation or from marginal disc herniation. Marked and irregular deformities also occur in the various epiphyseal dysplasias which may affect the spine (see Fig. 5.8). Long-standing osteoarthritis may also give rise to anterior deformities, possibly due to remodelling of the vertebral body. Such deformities are characterized by their uniform appearance.

FEMORAL NECK AND HEAD

The proximal femur has a distinctive pattern of trabecular architecture which is disturbed in the course of osteoporosis. Indeed, five anatomical groups of trabeculae can be defined which form the basis of the Singh score. The pattern of loss provides a semi-quantitative estimate of trabecular losses in osteoporosis which have proved to be of value in epidemiological studies. The six grades can be distinguished by the use of charts or reference radiographs (Fig. 5.9). Most patients with hip fractures have low scores, but many elderly individuals without hip fractures also have an abnormal score. The risk of hip fracture increases with decreasing score, an effect which is much more marked in the elderly (Wickham *et al.*, 1989).

CORTICAL BONE

There are two major characteristics of cortical bone loss in osteoporosis: thinning of the cortex and an increase in cortical porosity on X-rays. A number of quantitative techniques have been developed for their assessment. The size of some tubular bones increases with age. Thinning of the cortex thus represents an increase in net endocortical bone resorption. Cortical thickness has been assessed at many sites including the femur, but the site most frequently used is the metacar-

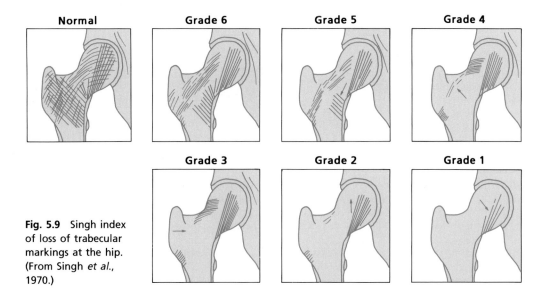

Fig. 5.9 Singh index of loss of trabecular markings at the hip. (From Singh *et al.*, 1970.)

pals (Exton-Smith *et al.*, 1969). Evaluation can be improved by magnification and the use of fine grain films.

Net endosteal resorption induces a scalloped appearance on the inner endocortical surface. Intracortical resorption is characterized by radiotranslucent streaks within cortical bone. The striations correspond to intracortical resorption bays and are more clearly visible using fine grain films or magnification techniques. As in the case of cortical width, these have been most carefully assessed at the metacarpal.

FOCAL OSTEOPOROSIS AND IMMOBILIZATION BONE LOSS

Radiographic features

Focal causes of osteoporosis and osteoporosis due to immobilization may induce rapid rates of bone loss and give rise to several characteristic radiographic features within a few weeks (Fig. 5.10). The most prominent is a loss of trabecular pattern, which may be particularly marked at the metaphyseal regions of long bones, especially in children

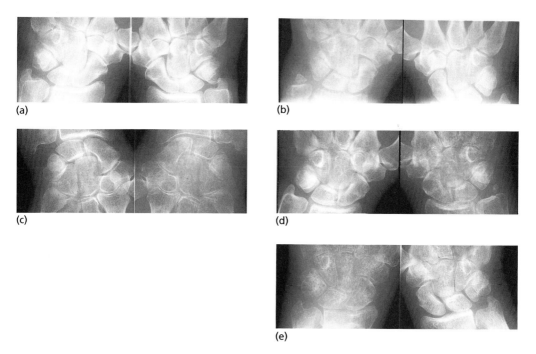

(a)

(b)

(c)

(d)

(e)

Fig. 5.10 Carpal radiographs taken 7 weeks after Colles' fracture showing various degrees and features of cancellous bone loss. Each panel shows the affected and unaffected side. (a) Shows a mild and diffuse loss of radiodensity. (b) Shows loss of density on the left and patchy radiotranslucency. (c) Shows generalized loss of density, patchy radiotranslucency and a loss of trabecular pattern. There is also a pencil-line appearance of the trabecular margin. (d) Shows more marked features with subarticular radiotranslucency. (e) Shows all features due to algodystrophy. (From Bickerstaff *et al.*, 1991a.)

139 / Assessment of bone mass

and young adults. In the carpals and tarsals a similar phenomenon occurs and may appear as a radiotranslucent margin beneath the cortical perimeter. Patchy loss of trabeculae also occurs. Semi-quantitative scales have been devised for each of these features. Contrary to popular belief, patchy radiotranslucency is not a feature solely of algodystrophy and occurs following simple immobilization or after a long bone fracture, though the features are less florid (Bickerstaff *et al.*, 1991b). As mentioned, transverse cortical striations may be visible on radiographs.

Algodystrophy

Bone biopsy

The indications for bone biopsy are relatively limited in routine clinical practice. However, bone biopsy may be the only way of excluding osteomalacia, and this is the most common clinical indication for biopsy outside the area of clinical research. The biochemical indices of osteomalacia are insensitive. Occasionally, unsuspected disease is first diagnosed at bone biopsy. Examples include masto-cytosis, myelomatosis, hyperparathyroidism, sarcoidosis, haemo-chromatosis and apudomas. Secondary causes are much more common in men and if a secondary cause is not apparent, bone biopsy is a valuable adjunct to investigation.

Evaluation of therapeutic intervention

Occasionally biopsy is utilized to evaluate the effects of therapeutic intervention. Examples include the response to vitamin D, the exclusion of complications arising from intervention such as osteomalacia due to treatment with fluoride or etidronate. Uncomplicated osteoporosis shows a great deal of heterogeneity in the disturbances of bone turnover (see Chapter 2), and some believe that the assessment of the rate of turnover is useful in targeting therapeutic strategies (see Chapter 7). If information on turnover alone is required, this can now be reasonably obtained either with the use of whole body retention of bisphosphonates or, more commonly, by the indirect biochemical indices.

Other laboratory assessments of skeletal status

Limited role of scintigraphy

Skeletal turnover (bone formation, mineralization and resorption) can be deduced from kinetic, histological or biochemical tests alone or in combination. Metabolic balance studies give an approximation of the net fluxes of calcium occurring across the skeleton. They do not, however, indicate the size of the unidirectional fluxes. This can be overcome to some extent by the use of tracer kinetic studies. For example, the rate of bone resorption can be calculated by the release of strontium or calcium isotopes from the skeleton, and together with balance studies, the resorption and formation rates can be calculated separately.

Scintigraphy has a limited role in the assessment of osteoporosis.

Uptake is increased acutely following fracture but in the case of vertebral fracture, increased uptake may persist for many months or even years. It is not known whether this is due to further subclinical fractures, but the high uptake should not be interpreted to denote that the fracture is recent. On the other hand, increased uptake in a patient known to have previously normal uptake more reliably indicates a new fracture or extension of a pre-existing fracture. Uptake is also increased in high-turnover states such as those occurring with rapid bone loss due to immobilization. This is most readily detected at metaphyseal sites of the appendicular skeleton where comparison between sides can be made.

There are many causes of increased scintigraphic uptake at the spine so that scans are best evaluated alongside appropriate skeletal radiographs.

MEASUREMENT OF HEIGHT

Arm span

Height loss is an obvious consequence of crush fracture and anterior wedging contributes to loss of height due to the kyphosis induced. Loss of height, however, also occurs with aging due to a decrease in the intervertebral disc spaces. There is a diurnal variation in height which decreases by approximately 1 cm towards the end of the day due to standing. Height and arm span are usually approximately equal in healthy individuals, so that measuring the arm span can give a useful indication of height loss. In measuring serial height it is important to use the same equipment which has been carefully standardized. Instruments such as the Harpenden stadeometer allow reproducible measurements and can be used to assess changes in height.

Clinical assessment of risk

Many studies have assessed the ability of clinical risk factors to predict low bone density or fractures. Some have advocated the use of such factors to identify high-risk individuals. In several instances, such as body weight or a premature menopause, there is a clear relationship to BMD or to other causes of osteoporotic fracture. The question arises whether the use of a panel of risk factors can be used in the assessment of individuals, particularly in women at the time of the menopause. Is is often said, for example, that the woman who

Risk factor score

will develop fractures is thin, smokes and drinks, and has a mother with osteoporosis. Several scores have been devised for clinical use to determine whether patients should receive treatment on this basis or be referred for further evaluation such as the measurement of bone density.

Many of the factors implicated in the causation or aggravation of bone loss are derived from observational studies (see Chapters 2 and 4) and the effect of confounding variables is uncertain. Good examples are parity, breast feeding and caffeine consumption, where the relationship is not consistently found. Apart from age, gender and race, many of the risk factors identified thus far, such as hyperparathyroidism, Cushing's disease, etc., are comparatively rare so that their impact value is correspondingly low for use in the general population though they are important aspects of case finding.

Diseases

Several studies have found that such information does not predict bone mass with sufficient precision to be useful in the management of individuals. For example, predictors of bone mass have been compared with the results actually measured. For femoral neck BMD, the best predictive model accounted for only 17% of the variability in bone mineral measurements at the hip and correctly classified only 65% of the perimenopausal women whose bone mass was in the lowest tertile (Slemenda et al., 1990). This is not adequate for patient care since bone mineral can be measured directly with less error of missclassification.

Poor predictive valve

An important predisposing factor is a prior fragility fracture. In one series, individuals with a high bone mass and the presence of a fragility fracture had a 10-fold increase in the risk of fracture over those in the lowest tertile of bone mineral (Ross et al., 1991).

Assessment of symptomatic patients

Postmenopausal and age-related bone loss are the most common forms of established osteoporosis seen in clinical practice. A detailed history is essential for diagnosis because it may suggest that the osteoporosis is secondary to other causes which occur relatively commonly, such as hyperthyroidism (either primary or iatrogenic), primary hyperparathyroidism, hypercorticolism, myeloma or osteomalacia. A family history and a history of fragility fractures may identify patients with mild osteogenesis imperfecta not previously diagnosed and which becomes a problem only after the menopause.

Detailed history

A thorough history also facilitates selection of appropriate baseline tests. Routine laboratory tests include full blood count and differential white cell count; measurement of the erythrocyte sedimentation rate, analysis of a fasting urine collection to measure indices of bone resorption (see Table 5.6); and determination of serum calcium, albumin, phosphorus, alkaline phosphatase, urea and creatinine. Serum calcium should be adjusted for fluctuations in albumin and serum phosphate and urine collections taken after an overnight fast. In asymptomatic postmenopausal disease, the results of routine laboratory tests are often normal and do not assess the extent or rate of bone loss or indicate the prognosis. Even in established but uncomplicated postmenopausal osteoporosis, the concentrations of serum calcium and inorganic phosphorus are usually within the normal range. Alkaline phosphatase levels may rise transiently for several months following a fracture. In the elderly we commonly measure

Routine laboratory tests

thyroid function and serum and urinary proteins since thyrotoxicosis and myeloma may be occult.

The diagnosis of osteoporosis is confirmed by the measurement of bone mineral mass. A low bone mass at first assessment gives no indication as to how or when bone loss occurred, or whether bone loss is continuing. The interpretation of density measurements with biochemical indices of skeletal turnover (see Table 5.6) are helpful for this reason to determine whether loss is currently occurring. Bone mass, particularly at the spine, often needs to be interpreted with appropriate X-rays to assess the possible contribution of osteo-arthrosis, apophyseal arthritis and vascular calcification.

Secondary osteoporosis

If bone loss secondary to conditions other than age-related and postmenopausal osteoporosis is suspected, additional tests may be required. In the absence of clinical signs of secondary causes a high index of suspicion is appropriate in all men, women under the age of 50 years and in the elderly, particularly those in institutionalized care to exclude osteomalacia. Additional investigations include the daily urinary excetion of calcium, serum calcidiol and PTH. The diagnosis of myelomatosis is usually straightforward and it should be suspected in adults over the age of 50 years who have severe osteo-porosis that is otherwise unexplained. Associated anaemia, proteinuria and a high sedimentation rate support the diagnosis which can be confirmed by protein electrophoresis on serum and urine. Rarely a non-secretory myeloma will require a bone marrow aspirate or needle biopsy.

Information on disturbances in calcium transport can be gained comparing the 24-hour and fasting excretion of calcium. A normal 24-hour calcium excretion in the presence of a high fasting urinary excretion suggests increased bone resorption. Increases in both suggest either massively increased bone resorption or that increased intesti-nal absorption is contributing as seen for example in sarcoidosis, vitamin D toxicity and hypercalciuric nephrolithiasis. Conversely, a low 24-hour urinary excretion suggests intestinal malabsorption of calcium and osteomalacia. The assessment of the manner in which calcium fluxes are disturbed at bone, gut and kidney is helpful in planning further investigations. The most useful and widely used tests are shown in Table 5A.

Risk factors

Men have a much higher likelihood of having secondary causes of osteoporosis than women since, in mature life, they have a greater bone mass, lose bone less rapidly and do not live as long as women. There have been relatively few studies of risk factors in men. For hip fracture, alcohol, smoking, a low body mass index, lack of physical activity and a propensity to falls have all been identified to carry a significantly increased risk. Similar factors have been identified for vertebral osteoporosis in men.

These risk factors are very similar to those identified for women, but the relative risk is in general higher than that found in women.

Table 5A Tests commonly used in the investigation of established osteoporosis

Test	Disorder
Gonadotrophins, especially follicle-stimulating hormone	Gonadal status
Thyroid function tests (T_3RU, T_4, thyroid-stimulating hormone)	Thyrotoxicosis
Scintigraphy	Carcinoma with skeletal metastases
Parathyroid hormone	Secondary hyperparathyroidism Osteomalacia Occult primary hyperparathyroidism
Marrow aspirate or needle biopsy	Myelomatosis
Bone biopsy	Osteomalacia, aluminium toxicity Mastocytosis Sarcoidosis
Gonadal hormones	Hypogonadism
Serum iron, ferritin	Haemochromatosis
Mantoux	Sarcoidosis
Serum calcitriol	Sarcoidosis and granulomatous disease
Serum calcidiol	Vitamin D deficiency or toxicity
Urinary phosphoethanolamine	Hypophosphatasia
Urinary free cortisol	Cushing's syndrome

Table 5B Causes of osteoporosis identified in 358 men with vertebral fracture. Combined data of Seeman *et al.* (1983), Francis *et al.* (1989), Allain *et al.* (1992) and a personal series of 115 patients

Cause or associated factor	Number	(%)
Unknown	181	(50.6)
Steroid treatment	59	(16.5)
Alcohol abuse	38	(10.7)
Hypogonadism	22	(6.1)
Gastric surgery	19	(5.3)
Osteogenesis imperfecta	11	(3.1)
Neoplasia	8	(2.2)
Anticonvulsants	7	(1.9)
Diabetes mellitus	4	(1.1)
Immobilization	2	(0.6)
Homocystinuria	2	(0.6)
Other*	5	(1.4)

* Includes liver disease, childhood rickets, mastocytosis, haemochromatosis (without liver disease).

A secondary cause for osteoporosis will be identified in approximately 50% of men with vertebral fracture. In these, exogenous use of corticosteroids, hypogonadism and high alcohol ingestion will account for more than half (Table 5B).

The detection of hypogonadism in men is not always clinically obvious. Where it occurs after puberty it may not be associated with testicular atrophy, and indeed testicular-deficient men may be capable of sexual function. In addition, patients may be reluctant to report a decrease in libido or they may accept this as a normal part of aging. For this reason serum testosterone as well as gonadotrophins should be measured routinely. It is important to note that serum testosterone may be normal. For example, normal values are found in a substantial minority of patients with Klinefelter's syndrome. If gonadotrophins are normal but testosterone decreased, assessment of pituitary function should be considered.

Where no secondary causes are found with an adequate laboratory-based investigation, a bone biopsy may be helpful in assessing the pathophysiology of the disorder as well as on occasion finding occult disease.

Assessment of asymptomatic patients

There are several disorders associated with a significantly increased

Table 5C Conditions in which bone mineral density measurement and intervention may be indicated

Women
Prolonged amenorrhoea
Anorexia nervosa
Exercise induced
Prolactinoma
Premature menopause (<45 years)
Idiopathic
Cancer chemotherapy
Pelvic irradiation
Late menses (>15 years)
Prolonged heparin infusion
Men and women
Primary hypogonadism
History of low energy-induced fracture
Chronic alcohol abuse
Incidental finding of osteopenia or vertebral fracture
History of prolonged immobilization
Certain diseases: e.g. long-standing thyrotoxicosis, chronic liver disease, Cushing's disease, hyperparathyroidism, chronic renal failure, haemochromatosis, mastocytosis, homocystinuria
Certain drugs: e.g., long-term corticosteroid use, anticonvulsants

risk of osteoporosis. Many of these provide indications for the assessment of BMD to diagnose osteoporosis or to assess future fracture risk. Examples are given in Table 5C. Since there are no clinical methods for accurately assessing fracture risk, the question arises whether measurements of bone mass should be used more widely in the community to identify apparently healthy individuals and to target treatment. In the absence of screening strategies most physicians interested in bone disease undertake the assessment of BMD where the outcome of the result would modify advice given to a patient. In the context of hormone replacement therapy (HRT), this might be whether a woman would be prepared to take HRT only where a reduction in bone density was shown to be unacceptably low.

The use of drug treatment to prevent osteoporosis is increasing in many countries as the awareness of osteoporosis grows. In the United Kingdom the use of calcium prescriptions has more than doubled in the past 4 years. In Europe, approximately 10% of women over the age of 50 years are taking or have taken bone-active drugs of one sort or another. In many instances this is non-targeted use for the prevention of osteoporosis, particularly with the use of calcium. If this money is to be spent, there is a strong case for redirecting it in a more appropriate manner by basing a decision whether or not to treat on the result of BMD assessments.

References

Allain T, Pitt P, Moniz C (1992) Osteoporosis in men. *BMJ*; **305**: 955–956.

Bickerstaff DR, O'Doherty DP, Kanis JA (1991a) Radiographic changes in algodystrophy of the hand. *J Hand Surg*; **16B**: 47–52.

Bickerstaff DR, O'Doherty DP, McCloskey EV, Hamdy NAT, Mian M, Kanis JA (1991b) Effects of amino-butylidene diphosphonate in hypercalcemia due to malignancy. *Bone*; **12**: 17–20.

Brown JP, Delmas PD, Malaval L, Edouard C, Chapuy MC, Meunier PJ (1984) Serum bone Gla-protein: a specific marker for bone formation in postmenopausal osteoporosis. *Lancet*; **i**: 1091–1093.

Cann CE (1988) Quantitative CT for determination of bone mineral density: a review. *Radiology*; **166**: 509–522.

Cosman F, Herrington B, Himmelstein S, Lindsay R (1991) Radiographic absorptiometry: a simple method for determining bone mass. *Osteoporosis Int*; **2**: 34–38.

Crilly RG, Jones MM, Horsman A, Nordin BEC (1980) Rise in plasma alkaline phosphatase at the menopause. *Clin Sci*; **58**: 341–342.

Cummings SR (1985) Are patients with hip fractures more osteoporotic? *Am J Med*; **78**: 487–494.

Cummings SR, Black DM, Nevitt MC *et al.* (1993) Bone density at various sites for prediction of hip fractures. *Lancet*; **341**: 72–75.

Dalen N, Hellstrom L, Jacobson B (1976) Bone mineral content and mechanical strength of the femoral neck. *Acta Orthop Scand*; **47**: 503–508.

Exton-Smith AN, Millard PH, Payne PR, Wheeler EF (1969) Method for measuring quantity of bone. *Lancet*; **ii**: 1153–1154.

Francis RM, Peacock M, Marshall DH, Horsman A, Aaron JE (1989) Spinal osteoporosis in men. *Bone Miner;* **5**: 347–357.

Hansen M, Overgaard K, Riis B, Christiansen C (1991) Role of peak bone mass and bone loss in postmenopausal osteoporosis: 12 year study. *BMJ;* **303**: 961–964.

Hui SL, Slemenda CS, Johnston CC (1988) Age and bone mass as predictors of fracture in a prospective study. *J Clin Invest;* **81**: 1804–1809.

Kanis JA (1991) *Pathophysiology and Treatment of Paget's Disease of Bone.* Martin Dunitz, London.

Kanis JA, Caulin F, Russell RGG (1983) Problems in the design of clinical trials in osteoporosis. In St J Dixon A, Russell RGG, Stamp TCB (eds). *Osteoporosis: A Multidisciplinary Problem. Royal Society of Medicine Int Cong Symp Series;* **55**: 205–222.

Kanis JA, McCloskey EV, Eyres KS, O'Doherty DV, Aaron JE (1990) Screening techniques in the evaluation of osteoporosis. In Drife JO, Studd JWW (eds). *HRT and Osteoporosis,* pp. 135–147. Springer Verlag, London.

Langton C, Palmer SB, Porter RW (1984) The measurement of broadband ultrasonic attenuation in cancellous bone. *Eng Med;* **13**: 89.

Mazess RB (1983) Errors in measuring trabecular bone by computed tomography due to marrow and bone composition. *Calcif Tissue Int;* **35**: 148.

Mazess RB, Wahner HM (1988) Nuclear medicine and densitometry. In Riggs BL, Melton III LJ (eds). *Osteoporosis, Aetiology, Diagnosis and Management,* pp. 251–295. Raven Press, New York.

McCloskey EV, Murray SA, Miller C *et al.* (1990) Broadband ultrasound attenuation in the os calcis: relationship to bone mineral at other skeletal sites. *Clin Sci;* **78**: 227–233.

McCloskey EV, Spector T, Eyres KS *et al.* (1993) Assessment of vertebral deformity – a method for use in population studies and clinical trials. *Osteoporosis Int;* **3**: 138–147.

Nilas L, Podenphant J, Riis BJ, Gotfredsen A, Christiansen C (1987) Usefulness of regional bone measurements in patients with osteoporotic fractures of the spine and distal forearm. *J Nucl Med;* **28**: 960–965.

Ohta H, Masuzawa T, Ikeda T, Suda Y, Makita K, Nozawa S (1992) Which is more osteoporosis-inducing, menopause or oophorectomy? *Bone Miner;* **19**: 273–285.

Palmer SB, Langton CM (1987) *Ultrasonic Studies of Bone.* Institute of Physics, Bristol.

Ross PD, Davis JW, Epstein RS, Wasnich RD (1991) Pre-existing fractures and bone mass predict vertebral fracture incidence in women. *Ann Intern Med;* **114**: 919–923.

Seeman E, Melton LJ, O'Fallon WM, Riggs BL (1983) Risk factors for spinal osteoporosis in men. *Am J Med;* **75**: 977–983.

Singh M, Nagrath AR, Malni PS (1970) Changes in trabecular pattern of the upper end of the femur as an index of osteoporosis. *J Bone Joint Surg;* **52A**: 457–467.

Slemenda CW, Hui SL, Longscope C, Wellman H, Johnston CC (1990) Predictors of bone mass in perimenopausal women: a prospective study of clinical data using photon absorptiometry. *Ann Intern Med;* **112**: 96–101.

Stepan JJ, Pospichal J, Presl J, Pacovsky V (1987) Bone loss and biochemical indices of bone remodelling in surgically induced postmenopausal women. *Bone;* **8**: 279–284.

Suman VJ, Atkinson EJ, O'Fallon WM, Black DM, Melton LJ (1993) A nomogram for predicting life-time hip fracture risk from radius bone mineral density and age. *Bone;* **14**: 843–846.

WHO (1994) Assessment of Osteoporotic Fracture Risk and its Role in Screening for Postmenopausal Osteoporosis. WHO Technical Report Series, Geneva.

Wickham CAC, Walsh K, Cooper C *et al.* (1989) Dietary calcium, physical activity and risk of hip fracture: a prospective study. *BMJ;* **299**: 889–992.

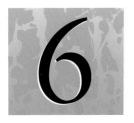

Prevention of osteoporosis from menarche to menopause

Strategies for prevention

Since osteoporosis – particularly postmenopausal osteoporosis – is widely prevalent, two distinct, but not mutually exclusive, preventive strategies can be envisaged. The first is to identify patients at particular risk and to offer an intervention. Examples include the identification of women with low bone density, patients likely to fall, or individuals with certain diseases. A second strategy is population based – the aim is to modify a risk factor within the general community. For example, if bone mineral density (BMD) were to be increased by 10% in the female population, this would decrease the risk of fragility fracture by 50% (Riggs & Melton, 1992). Such approaches might be directed at any stage or all stages of life.

POPULATION-BASED PREVENTION
Bone mass and rates of bone loss are continuously distributed in the population so that it is not possible to define precisely an individual with disease from the normal population. A number of risk factors have been identified which, if causally related and correctable, might have a significant impact on the burden of osteoporosis. The
Remedial factors more plausible remedial factors that have been proposed include a higher level of exercise, stopping smoking, a high calcium diet and the universal use of hormone replacement therapy (HRT) in postmenopausal women.

There are, however, several problems with this approach. The first is that not all these factors are necessarily causally related. These uncertainties exist for smoking and moderate alcohol consumption. A second problem relates to the ability to change lifestyle habits. Although several clinical trials have shown beneficial effects of exercise on bone mass or loss, it is likely that this type of intervention
Difficulties needs to be sustained for a lifetime. Bone loss is likely to occur as soon as this is stopped and, as is the case in many other branches of medicine, long-term compliance is likely to be very low. The relevance of exercise at the age of 40 years for 5 years to an individual aged 75 years is therefore questionable. In the case of exercise, the optimal

type and duration of exercise is also not known. This raises a third problem, namely that the value and feasibility of population-based programmes have never been evaluated. This consideration even applies to falls where intuition would dictate that attempts to prevent falls in the elderly would be of benefit. There is, however, currently no intervention proven to prevent the consequences of falls (Vetter *et al.*, 1992).

Low impact

A further problem relates to the impact of remedial factors on the frequency of fractures within a community. Despite the high prevalence of many of these factors, the increase in relative risk associated with each is relatively small (see Chapter 5). Thus, if all the risk factors that were identified for hip fracture were causal and could be reversed, the impact on the incidence of fracture would be less than 20%. In practice, the majority of risk factors are not feasibly remediable so that the impact would be very much lower.

The universal use of HRT is an approach which would have a much greater impact. It would likely decrease the burden of fractures by 50% or more in the female community. Apart from practicalities, the cost and the fact that most women do not continue to take HRT, problems arise in giving medicines with risks as well as benefits (reviewed on p. 152).

For all these reasons, population-based strategies of prevention are not presently feasible. Prevention is therefore more appropriately targeted to those segments of the community at high risk.

HIGH-RISK STRATEGY

In the context of osteoporosis (as distinct from fractures), prevention means the prevention of low bone mass. As in the case of a population strategy this could be directed to suitable individuals at any age. Since bone mass, at least up to the age of 75 years or so, is largely a function of peak bone mass, it could be argued that prevention should be directed towards the optimization of peak bone mass.

Irreversible factors

Unfortunately major contributions to peak bone mass (race and heritability) are unchangeable and the impact of other potential factors such as exercise and nutrition is of uncertain value. Moreover, there is little information available to know whether we might identify at adolescence or beforehand those destined to become osteoporotic and those who will fracture. Even if this were possible, it is unlikely that we would persuade 13 year olds to change their lifestyle or accept an intervention to prevent an uncertain event half a century later.

Lifestyle factors

Although the precise role of many lifestyle factors is conjectural, it is important to recognize that non-hormonal factors (i.e. non-oestrogen dependent) account for the large inter-regional differences in the incidence of osteoporosis, since these affect both men and women.

Similarly, the secular increase in the incidence of hip fracture observed in the United States and many European countries has been observed in men as well as women. These observations suggest that lifestyle factors are of great importance in determining bone mass and consequently the rates of osteoporotic fractures. The most plausible lifestyle factor is exercise, but it remains only a plausible hypothesis at present.

For all these reasons, the major thrust of preventative measures has been directed towards preventing bone loss that occurs in association with the menopause, on the diagnosis of disease or at the onset of immobilization. Interventions used are largely pharmacological. Of these, the greatest attention has been directed to the use of gonadal steroids.

HRT

The term hormone replacement treatment or therapy (HRT) is used generically to denote the use of oestrogens, either alone or in combination with progestogens. Where the distinction is necessary this is made explicit. The distinction is important since much of the thinking concerning the risks and benefits of HRT is significantly modulated by the choice of regimen. These considerations are least complicated in the case of the effects of HRT on osteoporotic fractures.

EFFECTS ON BONE

A great deal of prospective evidence indicates that the use of HRT will prevent bone loss at the menopause and indeed thereafter. Experience is greatest with conjugated oestrogens and long-term dose–response studies have been undertaken with this and some other preparations. The average bone-sparing dose of conjugated oestrogens is 0.625 mg daily and for oestradiol is 1–2 mg, and the response to lower doses is incomplete (Fig. 6.1; Christiansen et al., 1982). The skeletal effects of oestrogen do not depend on the route but rather the concentrations achieved (Reginster et al., 1992). Bone-sparing effects have been shown with transdermal and percutaneous routes.

On average, adequate doses of oestrogen prevent bone loss more or less completely, irrespective of when they are given in the course of osteoporotic bone loss. Long-term studies are limited to 10 years. On the basis of limited data, it is possible that bone loss recurs slowly after 7–8 years (Lindsay et al., 1980) which may relate to age-dependent losses or the incomplete effects of oestrogens to correct imbalances at remodelling sites. The difference in bone density between control and treated patients increases with time since bone loss continues in the absence of treatment.

Case-control and cohort studies consistently report that HRT

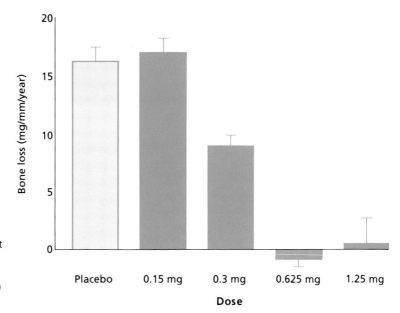

Fig. 6.1 Effects of placebo or conjugated oestrogens on the rate of bone loss assessed at the metacarpal according to dose over a 2-year interval. (From Lindsay *et al.*, 1984.)

Effect on fractures

Catch-up bone loss?

reduces the risk of hip fracture and forearm fractures in peri- or postmenopausal women. The pooled estimate of the relative risk of hip fracture comparing oestrogen users to non-users is 0.7 (95% confidence intervals, 0.6–0.79) (Grady *et al.*, 1992). Longer durations of exposure are associated with lower risks (Kanis *et al.*, 1992) suggesting that confounding factors between cases and controls is not the explanation for the difference. There are no prospective randomized studies examining the effects of oestrogen on hip fracture rates since prohibitively large numbers of patients would be required. Prospective studies have shown a significant difference in vertebral height or fractures between patients given oestrogens or placebo. Rates appear to decrease by 60–80%.

Progestogen therapy alone prevents bone loss and several studies have confirmed that combined oestrogen plus progestogen regimens prevent bone loss. Limited epidemiological data suggest that progestogens do not adversely alter the effect of oestrogens on hip fracture (Naessen *et al.*, 1990).

A major uncertainty is whether the effects of HRT persist or whether catch-up bone loss occurs (Pitt *et al.*, 1990). This is an important issue since HRT is commonly recommended for up to 10 years but the vast majority of fractures occur after the age of 70 years. Thus, a relatively short-term exposure at the menopause (e.g., 10 years) would only have significant beneficial effects on fracture risk if the effects were long lasting. Most direct evidence suggests that bone that has been preserved is not rapidly lost when oestrogen treatment is stopped, i.e., when bone loss recurs after stopping treatment it is at the same rate as it was just before therapy was instituted.

151 / Prevention

One early report which assessed bone density in oophorectomized women has been misinterpreted to indicate that catch-up bone loss occurred after stopping treatment, but this has not been observed in other studies. This has recently been confirmed in a 6-year follow-up of women after stopping HRT (Fig. 6.2). This suggests that the effects of the menopause persist for at least 6 years, i.e., the amount of bone saved during oestrogen therapy is saved for at least 6 years and probably much longer.

Hip fracture risk

In contrast, several epidemiological case-control studies have shown that the protective effects of oestrogens on the risk of hip fracture persist into extreme old age, but the relative risk is less than that of individuals more recently exposed to oestrogens (Law et al., 1991). A persistent effect of oestrogens is plausible and supported by the prospective evidence. The question arises why there is an apparent discrepancy between the conclusions derived from epidemiological research and clinical research. The epidemiological data are retrospective case-control or observational studies in the elderly which do not take account of deaths since those who die are not available for investigation.

Biases

In view of the increased comorbidity and the higher death rate of osteoporotic individuals, it is to be expected that the apparent protective effect of oestrogen on hip fracture risk would be less apparent the more elderly the population. This suggests that the case for a transient effect of oestrogens is weak but is an important area for further research.

NON-SKELETAL RISKS AND BENEFITS

A detailed assessment of the non-skeletal risks and benefits of HRT is beyond the scope of this chapter and is the subject of several reviews (Mack & Ross, 1990; Daly et al., 1991; Jacobs & Loeffler, 1992). Notwithstanding, it is inappropriate to ignore the risks and

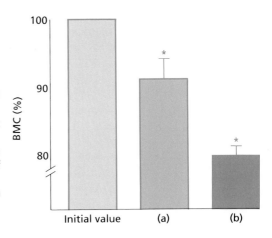

Fig. 6.2 Bone mineral content (BMC) at the distal radius (expressed as a percentage of initial value ±SEM) in 68 women taking hormone replacement therapy (HRT) for 4 years followed by no treatment for 6 years (a) and in 177 women given no treatment for 10 years (b). Note that values of the treated women lie midway between starting values and values after no treatment, indicating a persistent effect of earlier HRT. * = $P < 0.001$. (From Stevenson et al., 1992.)

benefits of intervention since they impact critically onto strategies for treatment.

Coronary heart disease

The incidence of coronary heart disease is relatively low in premenopausal women, but the differences between the sexes decrease progressively with age. This has been attributed to oestrogen deficiency at the menopause but in England the change in risk with age affects men rather than women. Irrespective of whether the menopause might protect males, the relationship between cardiovascular disease and loss of ovarian function is well established in many ways (Fig. 6.3) but the mechanism is not.

Oestrogen and heart disease

Systematic reviews of the literature reveal fairly consistent evidence that oestrogen therapy decreases the risk of coronary heart disease by about 30–50%. The dose of oestrogen used in most of the studies indicating protection from coronary heart disease is 0.625–1.25 mg/day of oral conjugated oestrogen. There are insufficient data to determine the optimum duration of oestrogen treatment to prevent coronary heart disease. All these data are derived from observational studies that are subject to bias. Some of the apparent protective effects of oestrogen might be due to the fact that more healthy women take oestrogen.

Lipids

Serum lipoprotein concentrations are a strong risk factor for coronary heart disease in women. Oestrogen therapy has been shown to reduce total serum cholesterol and low-density lipoprotein (LDL) cholesterol and to increase serum high-density lipoprotein (HDL) cholesterol in a dose-dependent fashion. Several progestogens attenuate the beneficial effect of oestrogen on lipoproteins, raising the concern that the addition of progestogen might negate some of the cardioprotective effects of oestrogens (Bush *et al.*, 1987). The extent to which the

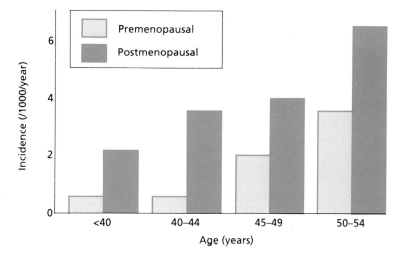

Fig. 6.3 Incidence of cardiovascular disease in women according to age and menopausal status. (From Kannel *et al.*, 1976.)

beneficial effect of oestrogen on lipoproteins is reversed depends on the type, dose and duration of progesterone use. The C-21 progestogens such as medroxyprogesterone acetate have fewer side effects and less unfavourable effects on lipoproteins than the C-19 progestins. In addition, the intermittent use of progestogens has few long-term consequences on lipid profiles in that the acute changes are ill-sustained.

Changes in lipoproteins may not be the sole mechanism by which oestrogens reduce cardiovascular risk. Several experiments on monkeys and rabbits fed atherogenic diets have found that oestrogen protected against the development of atherosclerosis. The combination of oestradiol and progesterone had no effect on HDL and total cholesterol, but appeared to protect against the development of atherosclerosis as effectively as oestrogen alone. Moreover, several clinical studies have determined the effect of oestrogens on coronary heart disease risk after adjusting for changes in lipids. Less than half of the reduction in risk by oestrogen treatment was accounted for by changes in lipids (Bush et al., 1987).

These observations suggest that if progestogens have adverse effects on coronary heart disease, they are likely to be small, and much smaller than the beneficial effects of oestrogens. Only two studies have directly assessed the effects of treatment with oestrogen plus a progestogen on cardiovascular risk in women. One small randomized controlled trial found a substantial but non-significant reduction in relative risk. A larger study suggested that the degree of protection appears to be as great as that observed for women taking oestrogen alone (Persson et al., 1990). These data suggest that the risk for coronary heart disease is reduced among women taking oestrogen plus a progestogen, but there are inadequate data to determine if this protective effect is of the same magnitude as that of unopposed oestrogen.

The effects of HRT on ischaemic heart disease impact significantly onto strategies for screening women at the menopause for fracture risk. The greater the benefit of HRT on cardiovascular risk, the poorer the case for targeting intervention on the basis of bone mineral measurements. In one study, more quality of life years would be saved by the universal use of HRT at the menopause (and the cost less) than with a programme of HRT use in high-risk women identified by screening for BMD (17% of the population, 15-year treatment) if the risk for coronary artery disease decreased by 25% or more in treated women.

Endometrial cancer

The long-term use of unopposed oestrogens increases the risk of endometrial cancer. Pooled estimates of relative risk of endometrial cancer in women who have ever used oestrogen compared to those who have never used oestrogen is 2.4 (Grady et al., 1992). The effect is dose dependent and the risk increases with increasing duration of oestrogen use. The effects on mortality are less secure. Histological, clinical and epidemiological studies suggest that the addition of a progestogen to the oestrogen regimen prevents the increase in endometrial cancer risk provided that the dose and schedule of progestogen therapy is adequate to prevent endometrial hyperplasia.

Breast cancer

No consistent effect

The view that oestrogen therapy is associated with an increased risk of breast cancer is plausible. A delayed menarche or early menopause is associated with a lower risk. A lower risk is also reported in former athletes, perhaps related to leanness and peripheral metabolism of oestrogen. There have been at least 24 case-control studies of oestrogen therapy and breast cancer risk since 1970, but the findings are inconsistent. Three recently published analyses of these studies found no increased risk for breast cancer in women who took oestrogen. Studies that have evaluated the effect of long-term oestrogen use have also had conflicting results. Many show a small increase in risk among women who have taken oestrogen for the longest duration, whereas others do not. A recent meta-analysis suggested that 15 years of oestrogen use might increase the risk of breast cancer by as much as 30% (relative risk 1.3, 95% confidence intervals 1.2–1.6) (Steinberg et al., 1991). On the other hand, an increase in mortality from breast cancer in women taking HRT has not been

HRT may accelerate presentation of breast cancer

shown. It seems plausible that the propensity to develop breast cancer is established in early life and that HRT might accelerate its presentation.

It is notable that in healthy women the risk of breast cancer increases progressively with age, but that the rate of increase is attenuated at about the time of the menopause. Thus, the increased relative risk of breast cancer in the treated population may reflect no more than the continuing oestrogen status of such women. This notion is consistent with the observed increase in risk of breast cancer in women with a late menopause. Evidence in women concerning the effects of oestrogen plus progestogen is too limited to estimate their effects on breast cancer risk.

Cerebrovascular disease

Stroke

There is some evidence that oestrogen decreases the risk of stroke, but there is no information on the effect of oestrogen plus progestogen regimens on stroke risk in women.

Overall risks and benefits

Selection biases

Most of the information on the risks and benefits of HRT have been derived from observational studies. Women who elect to take HRT are known to differ in many important respects from those who do not, e.g., they are generally better educated, exercise more, have a 50% lower risk of suicide and lower morbidity and mortality rates. It is only possible to adjust for known or quantifiable biases. In addition, there is likely to be a significant bias in published literature in that negative studies are less likely to be accepted. This may result in an overestimate of both the apparent risks and apparent benefits.

With all these limitations, a number of studies have assessed the overall benefits and risks of HRT (e.g., Daly *et al.*, 1991), but are beyond the scope of this review. Under most assumptions, however, **Benefits outweigh risks** the perceived benefits outweigh the risks, both in terms of mortality (Table 6.1) and morbidity. Because of the multiplicity of effects of HRT, it is apparent that the gains will differ according to the type of population exposed. For example, women with a hysterectomy have no need for combined preparations and therefore are not exposed to any potential risks of added progestogens. Moreover, women with a high risk of coronary heart disease may have more to gain in terms of morbidity and life-expectancy than women at risk from hip fracture. These considerations suggest that hormone therapy should probably **Targeting treatment** be recommended for women who have had a hysterectomy and those with a high risk for coronary heart disease. In women with coronary heart disease who have not had a hysterectomy, treatment with oestrogen alone is likely to increase life-expectancy but also increase the risk of endometrial cancer. To prevent this risk, unacceptable to physicians in some countries, the addition of progestogens to the oestrogen regimen is preferred. Even if the added progestogen reduces the benefits of oestrogen on coronary heart disease by one-third,

Table 6.1 The net change in life expectancy for a 50-year-old woman from the United States treated with long-term hormone replacement therapy (15 years) according to the presence of risk factors. E denotes treatment with oestrogen alone, E + P the combination with progestogens. (From Grady *et al.*, 1992)

	Life expectancy (years)	Change in life expectancy (years)		
		E	E + P*	E + P†
No risk factors	82.8	+0.8	+0.9	+0.1
With hysterectomy	82.8	+1.0	—	—
History of coronary heart disease	76.0	+1.8	+1.8	+0.9
Risk of coronary heart disease	79.6	+1.3	+1.4	+0.5
At risk of breast cancer	81.8	+0.4	+0.4	−1.0
At risk of hip fracture	82.4	+0.9	+1.0	+0.2

* Assumes that P decreases all risk of endometrial cancer.
† Assumes that P additionally decreases cardiovascular benefit (relative risk = 0.8) by one-third, increases the relative risk of breast cancer from 1.3 to 2.0, but without effect on fracture frequency (relative risk = 0.7).

women with coronary heart disease will still benefit substantially, increasing average life-expectancy by about a year.

Management of the menopause

The management of the menopause is more than the prescription for HRT. A detailed account is beyond the scope of this book but there are several aspects that are important to consider. The focus of management is still the symptomatic relief of acute symptoms but in recent years has begun to embrace the prevention of its long-term complications such as osteoporosis and cardiovascular disease. Thus the assessment of patients may include the assessment of acute symptoms, as well as assessments of risks for cardiovascular disease and for osteoporosis. The dose and duration of use of HRT or other interventions depends upon the various aims of treatment.

Aims of management

ACUTE MENOPAUSAL SYMPTOMS
Acute menopausal symptoms (see Chapter 2) are common. Management generally involves a combination of counselling, HRT or non-hormonal drug therapy.

Relief of oestrogen-deficiency symptoms

Oestrogen replacement therapy will relieve or modify all the symptoms that are due to oestrogen deficiency; in the case of hot flushes, it is effective in 95% of women. Hot flushes and night sweats improve within 2 weeks of starting treatment, although relief from other symptoms may take longer. Maximum therapeutic response to any particular dosage is usually achieved within 3 months. If symptoms are not adequately controlled, then the dose may be increased or the patient changed to an alternative preparation. The severity of menopausal symptoms is thought to be related to the fluctuations in endogenous gonadal status. This gradually decreases over several years. For this reason, treatment is commonly stopped after a few years and symptoms are less likely to recur.

Symptoms related to fluctuations in gonadal status

Progestogens

Progestogens (e.g., norethisterone 5 mg/day) can be effective in controlling hot flushes and night sweats and are also useful in cases where oestrogen therapy is contraindicated. Hypnotics, sedatives and tranquillizers are widely prescribed and may improve hot flushes but do not relieve other menopausal symptoms. Indeed, they can sometimes add to a patient's feeling of lethargy. Water-soluble lubricants or vaginal moisturizers can relieve vaginal dryness and may reduce dyspareunia, where the atrophic changes are minimal.

PREVENTION OF OSTEOPOROSIS

Oestrogen replacement therapy effectively prevents bone loss in postmenopausal women. This arrest of bone loss will last as long as oestrogen treatment continues, at least up to the age of 70 years and possibly beyond. When oestrogen treatment

the case of cardiovascular disease, there is little evidence that these should be considered as contraindications.

There are, however, several disorders where a more careful assessment is appropriate (Table 6A). In a few individuals, blood pressure may increase markedly so this should be measured before and after the start of treatment. If hypertension occurs, it is reversed when treatment is stopped. Similarly, oestrogens may induce or exacerbate migraine in a susceptible minority which reverses when treatment is stopped.

Clotting disorders

In the case of a history of deep venous thrombosis or pulmonary embolism, it is important to distinguish events which occurred without any risk factor and may be associated with abnormalities in coagulation, from those which have arisen after trauma such as childbirth and pelvic surgery. Patients with spontaneous thrombosis or those occurring during pregnancy or on the contraceptive pill, should not be given oestrogens unless abnormalities of coagulation or fibrinolysis have been excluded.

Diabetes

Diabetes is not an absolute contraindication but glucose levels should be monitored and insulin dosage adjusted if necessary. Glucose tolerance is not adversely affected in otherwise healthy women. There is some epidemiological evidence that the risk of gallstones is increased in women given HRT. HRT should therefore be prescribed with caution and a non-oral route may be preferable in such patients as well as those with mild liver disease and previous liver disease.

Endometriosis

Endometriosis can present a difficult problem of management since oestrogens may reactivate the disease, even in patients where there

Table 6A Relative and absolute contraindications for hormone replacement therapy

Relative contraindications
Uncontrolled hypertension
Migraine
Previous deep venous thrombosis or pulmonary embolism
Diabetes
Pre-existing gallstones
Mild liver disease
Endometriosis
Fibroids
Previous breast cancer
Endometrial cancer
Absolute contraindications
Active endometrial or breast cancer
Pregnancy
Undiagnosed abnormal vaginal bleeding
Severe active liver disease
? Melanoma

has been apparent surgical removal of all affected tissue. The risk, however, is small. Unopposed oestrogen therapy (oestrogen without a progestogen) can be given to women who have had a hysterectomy and bilateral salpingo-oophorectomy with complete excision of all the endometriotic tissue. Otherwise, it may be preferable to use a combined (with progestogen) regimen and monitor treatment by regular pelvic examination at 6-monthly or yearly intervals. Fibroids may also become enlarged with oestrogen therapy and cause heavy or painful withdrawal bleeds. The patient should obviously be advised of this and treatment monitored by regular pelvic examination.

Fibroids

There are no available data to indicate that the risk of breast cancer recurrence is increased in patients on oestrogen treatment. The major reason for this, however, is that such women have never systematically been prescribed oestrogen therapy. Many regard previous breast cancer as an absolute contraindication to oestrogen therapy or at least recommend a period of a few years before treatment is started. Others, including ourselves, consider that where quality of life is severely impaired by menopausal symptoms or the risk of fractures is very high, such patients, after careful counselling, may be offered oestrogen therapy, perhaps in combination with tamoxifen.

Breast cancer

Management of patients with endometrial cancer depends on the extent of the invasion of the myometrium, histology and whether or not there is cervical and uterine involvement. Some are given oestrogen or progestogens with stage I endometrial cancer but it is a controversial issue.

There remain a few absolute contraindications to oestrogen therapy. These include active endometrial or breast cancer, pregnancy, undiagnosed abnormal vaginal bleeding and severe active liver disease with abnormal liver function tests. Melanoma may recur more rapidly during pregnancy and HRT for this reason is usually avoided.

Absolute contraindications

TYPES OF OESTROGEN THERAPY

So-called natural oestrogens are utilized for HRT. These include 17β-oestradiol and its derivatives, oestrone, oestriol and conjugated equine oestrogens isolated from pregnant mares' urine. Synthetic oestrogens such as mestranol and ethinyloestradiol are not commonly used. In women with a hysterectomy, oestrogens may be given continuously. Oestrogen replacement therapy can be administered by a variety of routes. The most commonly used are the oral route and transcutaneous regimens which are convenient, inexpensive and can be easily stopped.

Opposed oestrogen therapy

Many physicians prefer to use opposed regimens in women with intact uteri. Others monitor endometrial hyperplasia by non-invasive techniques such as ultrasound. After the progestogen is stopped, women experience a withdrawal bleed and the return of monthly periods is the most common reason for non-compliance among women.

Progestogens used in HRT can be classified as C-21 derivatives (such as norethisterone) and C-19 progestogens (such as medroxy-progesterone acetate). The C-21 progestogens are generally used for HRT because they have fewer adverse lipid effects but the doses of norethisterone used (generally 1 mg) have no appreciable effects. Most combined oestrogen/progestogen products in clinical use contain 10, 12 or 13 days progestogen for each 28 days of oestrogen. Cyclical opposed oestrogen regimens may be fixed, in which commercially available preparations, often in one tablet, contain a daily dose of oestrogen which is given for 21−28 days and progestogens for the last 10−13 days. Others prefer to tailor the dose and duration of hormones to the individual.

Side effects of progestogens vary considerably depending on dose duration and andogenicity of the progestogen. Side effects that are commonly experienced by women receiving cyclical progestogens are fluid retention or 'bloating' which may be relieved by changing to another progestogen, mastalgia, headache, mood changes and acne.

Side effects of oestrogens also include fluid retention, breast tenderness and headaches but they are less common than after the use of progestogens. Additional side effects include nausea, leg cramps, dyspepsia and heavy withdrawal bleeds. In most patients body weight falls although the perception in patients may differ. Long-term treatment decreases total fat mass and preserves this in a gynaecoid rather than android distribution.

Combined continuous regimens

In many countries, combined continuous oestrogen and progestogen regimens are available. They are particularly suitable for postmenopausal rather than perimenopausal women in whom withdrawal bleeds are not tolerated. These regimens generally do not induce cyclical bleeding and suppress endometrial proliferation. In about a quarter of women, irregular bleeding may occur, particularly after the onset of treatment. This can be minimized by increasing the dose of progestogen where oestrogen and progestogen are being used separately.

Adverse lipid profiles have not been observed. HDL increases and LDL decreases and total cholesterol decreases. No change has been observed in serum triglycerides and VLDL. A commonly used regimen of 2 mg 17β-oestradiol combined with 1 mg norethisterone prevents bone loss without adverse effects on lipid metabolism (Fig. 6.5).

Other routes of administration

With the transdermal delivery system, oestradiol is released continuously into the bloodstream from a patch placed on the skin. Side effects are few; the most frequent are headache and skin reactions at

the site of application. Transdermal delivery bypasses the liver and

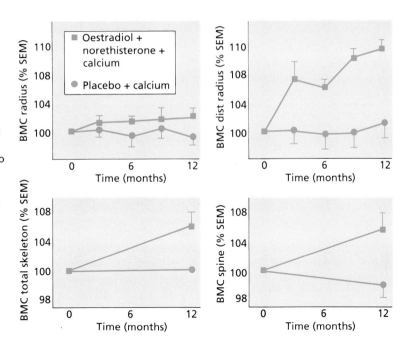

Fig. 6.5 Effects of combined continuous oestradiol (2 mg daily) and norethisterone (1 mg daily) or placebo on measurements of bone mineral content (BMC) in women with osteoporosis. Both groups additionally received 500 mg calcium daily. Values are expressed as percentage of initial values ±SEM. (From Christiansen & Riis, 1990.)

the effects on lipoproteins may not be as pronounced by this route as with oral oestrogens. It may be advantageous in patients with mild liver disease or gallstones.

Implants

Implants of oestriol are given as a pellet implanted into the subcutaneous fatty layers. It is most frequently used at time of surgery in women undergoing oophorectomy or hysterectomy. It is more suitable for hysterectomized women and women with a uterus should take progestogens.

Topical use

Topical oestrogen vaginal creams, pessaries and tablets have a potent local action and effectively relieve vaginal dryness and atrophic vaginitis. The rate of absorption of oestrogens from the vagina varies considerably and cyclical progestogens may be needed.

OTHER TREATMENT REGIMENS

Testosterone

Libido

Loss of libido in some women can often be improved by oestrogen therapy. If loss of libido persists when all other menopausal symptoms have cleared, libido may be increased after testosterone implants: the usual dose is 100 mg repeated every 4–6 months but half the dose can be used if side effects occur. Side effects are rare; occasional hirsutism can be managed by withholding further implants or reducing the dose.

Tibolone

Tibolone is a synthetic analogue of the gonadal steroids with combined oestrogenic, progestogenic and androgenic properties. It binds preferentially with oestrogen receptors whereas its metabolites have greater affinity for progesterone and androgen receptors. It is closely related to the anabolic steroids but is considered here since it is increasingly used in perimenopausal women. It prevents oestrogen-deficiency bone loss, at least at the metacarpal, is effective in controlling hot flushes and sweats, and can also improve mood and libido. It does not cause endometrial proliferation at a dose of 2.5 mg/day and there is, therefore, no withdrawal bleed. The long-term effects of tibolone on cardiovascular morbidity have not been evaluated but it decreases both HDL and LDL and may increase insulin resistance. Other anabolic steroids are reviewed in Chapter 8.

Tamoxifen and raloxifene

Several antioestrogens, including tamoxifen and raloxifene, delay bone loss in postmenopausal women. Tamoxifen may accelerate skeletal losses before the menopause. Raloxifene is currently being developed as a therapeutic alternative to HRT since it has few if any effects on the endometrium.

COMPLIANCE

Problems with compliance

Despite much public awareness concerning the problems of osteoporosis and the effects of HRT on its natural history, the major problems with HRT are the reluctance of women to take it and the reluctance to take it for sufficient periods of time to have significant effects on fracture risk. The uptake of HRT in the United Kingdom is approximately 10% of postmenopausal women. Higher uptake occurs in Denmark and the United States but lower rates are seen in other European countries (Kanis et al., 1992).

Virtually no information is available concerning 5–10-year compliance rates, which is the duration of use that is usually recommended for the prevention of fractures. In one study, set in the context of screening, 63% of those taking HRT were compliant at 3 months and 53% were compliant at 12 months (D. Purdie, personal communication 1992).

Benefits of HRT

The perception of the benefits of HRT is changing rapidly and the growth of HRT prescriptions is increasing in many countries. Nevertheless, the majority of women at risk do not receive HRT for sufficient periods of time to make a significant impact on fracture risk. For this reason there has been much interest in the use of alternative agents for the prevention of bone loss at the menopause.

Non-HRT methods of prevention

Other agents available

Alternative therapies for the prevention of osteoporosis have been studied in less depth than HRT. Of the many agents known to affect bone metabolism, further consideration is worthy of the calciums, calcitonins and the bisphosphonates, all of which are available and are increasingly being used. They have all been tested in the setting of prevention and have been shown to prevent or at least to decrease the rate of bone loss in postmenopausal women. The evidence for their efficacy and the manner of their use is detailed in Chapter 7. The trophic effects of exercise on the skeleton have stimulated the use of many exercise regimens in order to prevent bone loss.

Exercise

Many animal studies indicate that bone is responsive to strain. For this and other reasons (see Chapters 3 and 4) many have advocated the use of exercise as a method of preventing osteoporosis. The available evidence would suggest that weight-bearing exercises are the more effective, but the threshold of exercise, its type, degree and periodicity that are optimal for bone mass are not known. The bulk of evidence is from observational studies and is almost certainly confounded by selection factors. Thus, more reasonable evidence for an effect of exercise should be derived from prospective studies. Though there are prospective studies reported, not all are randomized, which increases the difficulty in assessing the benefits. A prospective study in premenopausal women has shown an effect of weight-lifting exercises which resulted in an increase in lumbar bone mineral of less than 1% in 1 year (Gleeson *et al.*, 1990). Another study of weight training involving loading of the spine showed no increase in lumbar bone mineral. Indeed, it decreased compared to the controls (Fig. 6.6). Exercise regimens have also been tested in postmenopausal women and in men. In one controlled study, lumbar bone mineral increased by 3.5% in 8 months. Most other studies have shown less marked changes and, in some, bone loss. One study in postmenopausal women found no effect of walking on lumbar bone mineral, but

Weight-bearing exercises

Inconsistent effects

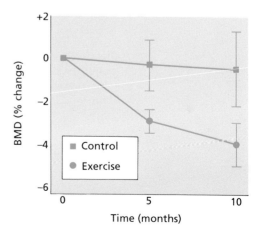

Fig. 6.6 The effect of a weight training regimen on bone mineral density of the lumbar spine (mean ± SEM) in 10 premenopausal women. Changes were significantly different from initial values after 9 months in women taking exercise ($P < 0.01$) and significantly different from controls ($P < 0.05$). (From Rockwell *et al.*, 1990.)

small increases occurred in another when resistance exercises were done.

A meta-analysis would undoubtedly come to the conclusion that exercise, particularly strength and aerobic regimens, increased bone mineral, but despite the effect of exercise, there are several factors to consider in its practical use. The first is that exercise regimens tend to increase lean body mass and decrease fat mass. These changes introduce errors of accuracy into the sequential determination of bone density with absorptiometry techniques and may overestimate the apparent effects of treatment at some sites (see Chapter 5). Thus, the effects are modest and are likely to persist only for the duration of exposure to exercise. It is difficult to change the habits of a lifetime and the dropout rate of organized regimens is very high (Glesson *et al.*, 1990) even where enthusiasm borders on evangelical. For this reason, the impact of exercise regimens is likely to be small. In addition, and as reviewed previously, exercise does not prevent bone loss due to oestrogen deficiency. The most elegant example is seen in exercise-induced amenorrhoea, where bone loss occurs despite adequate nutrition and high levels of exercise. Finally, intensive exercise is not without risks, including stress fracture and osteoporosis in the presence or absence of overt gonadal failure. The cardiovascular mortality is low and estimated at 1/116 000 exercise hours.

These considerations suggest a rather limited role for load-bearing exercise in the prevention of osteoporosis at the menopause. Quite different considerations apply to isometric exercises in patients with established osteoporosis (see Chapter 8).

Difficulties

Increase lean body mass

Exercise-induced amenorrhoea

References

Bush TL, Barrett-Connon E, Cowan LD *et al.* (1987) Cardiovascular mortality and noncontraceptive use of oestrogen in women: results from the Lipid Research Clinics Program follow-up study. *Circulation*; **75**: 1102−1109.

Christiansen C, Riis BJ (1990) Five years with continuous combined oestrogen/progestogen therapy. Effects of calcium metabolism, lipoproteins, and bleeding pattern. *Br J Obstet Gynaecol*; **97**: 1087−1092.

Christiansen C, Christensen MS, Larsen NE, Transbol I (1982). Pathophysiology mechanisms of estrogen effect on bone metabolism. Dose response relationships in early postmenopausal women. *J Clin Endocrinol Metab*; **55**: 1124−1130.

Daly E, Roche M, Barlow D, Gray A, McPherson K, Vessey M (1991) Hormone replacement therapy in the menopause: an analysis of benefits, risks and costs. Report to the Department of Health, UK.

Gleeson PB, Protas E, LeBlanc A, Schneider VS, Evans HJ (1990) Effects of weight lifting on bone mineral density in premenopausal women. *J Bone Miner Res*; **5**: 153−158.

Grady D, Rubin SM, Petitti *et al.* (1992) Hormone therapy to prevent disease and prolong life in postmenopausal women. *Ann Intern Med*; **117**: 1016−1037.

Jacobs HS, Loeffler FE (1992) Postmenopausal hormone replacement therapy. *BMJ*; **305**: 1403−1408.

Kanis JA, Johnell O, Gullberg B *et al.* (1992) Evidence for the efficacy of bone active drugs in the prevention of hip fracture. *BMJ*; **305**: 1124–1128.

Kannel WB, Hjortland MC, McNamara PM, Gordon T (1976) Menopause and risk of cardiovascular disease: The Framingham Study. *Ann Intern Med*; **85**: 447–452.

Law MR, Wald NJ, Meade TW (1991) Strategies for prevention of osteoporosis and hip fracture. *BMJ*; **303**: 453–459.

Lindsay R, Hart DM, Forrest C, Baird C (1980) Prevention of spinal osteoporosis in oophorectomised women. *Lancet*; **2**: 1151–1154.

Lindsay R, Hart DM, Clark DM (1984) The minimum effective dose of estrogen for prevention of postmenopausal bone loss. *Obstet Gynecol*; **63**: 754–763.

Mack RM, Ross PK (1990) A current perception of HRT risks and benefits. In DeLuca HF, Mazess R (eds). *Osteoporosis: Physiological Basis, Assessment and Treatment*, pp. 161–178. Elsevier Science, Amsterdam.

Naessen T, Persson I, Adami H-O, Bergstrom R, Bergkvist L (1990) Hormone replacement therapy and the risk for first hip fracture. *Ann Intern Med*; **113**: 95–103.

Persson I, Falkeborn M, Lithell H (1990) The effect of myocardial infarction (MI) risk of estrogens and estrogen-progestin combinations. In *Sixth International Congress on the Menopause*, p. 223. The Parthenon Publishing Group, Bangkok.

Pitt FA, Lloyd-Jones M, Brazier JE *et al.* (1990) The costs and benefits of screening and preventing post-menopausal osteoporosis in Trent Region. Report of the Trent Osteoporosis Working Group 1990. Trent Health, UK.

Reginster JY, Sarlet N, Deroisy R *et al.* (1992) Minimal levels of serum estradiol prevent postmenopausal bone loss. *Calcif Tissue Int*; **51**: 340–343.

Riggs BL, Melton LJ (1992) The prevention and treatment of osteoporosis. *N Engl J Med*; **327**: 620–627.

Rockwell JC, Sorensen AM, Baker S *et al.* (1990) Weight training decreases vertebral bone density in premenopausal women: a prospective study. *J Clin Endocrinol Metab*; **71**: 988–993.

Steinberg K, Thacker S, Smith S *et al.* (1991) A meta-analysis of the effect of estrogen replacement therapy on the risk of breast cancer. *JAMA*; **265**: 1985–1990.

Stevenson JC, Kanis JA, Christiansen C (1992) Bone density measurement. *Lancet*; **339**: 370–371.

Vetter NJ, Lewis PA, Ford D (1992) Can health visitors prevent fractures in elderly people? *BMJ*; **304**: 888–890.

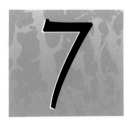

Treatment of generalized osteoporosis with inhibitors of bone resorption

Geographical differences in use

A surprisingly large number of bone-active agents have been used in osteoporosis but there is a great deal of heterogeneity in their use. For example, fluoride is widely used in France and Germany, but not licensed for use in the United States or United Kingdom. Calcitonin is available in all countries but more than 70% of the world sales are confined to Japan and Italy. The wide difference in prescribing habits poses problems for describing the treatment of osteoporosis in a manner appropriate for all countries.

Many agents are used in the treatment of osteoporosis (Table 7A). They can be broadly but inaccurately classed as inhibitors of bone turnover or stimulators of bone formation, but all act at least in part by altering the turnover of bone. Of these, the most is known about the effects of calcium, calcitonins and bisphosphonates on the turnover of bone, and skeletal mass and fracture. These agents are considered in this chapter, but it is relevant to consider the general effects of such interventions on bone before describing their individual effects.

Therapeutic modulation of bone turnover and balance

Decrease in bone turnover

Several inhibitors of bone turnover (also used in prophylaxis) appear to decrease the rate of bone loss, but may not prevent it entirely. The reason for this probably relates to their effect on bone remodelling. Thus, at each remodelling site a finite volume of bone is resorbed and in osteoporosis a somewhat lesser amount is formed. When bone turnover alone is decreased, the number of remodelling sites also decreases, but the imbalance between formation and resorption at each remodelling site may persist. Thus, if bone turnover is decreased by 50% bone loss would be reduced from, say, 2% to 1% per annum.

In contrast to this schema, many observations have shown that the inhibitors of bone turnover increase skeletal mass in osteoporosis. Although treatment is associated with an increase in skeletal mass, this is modest (2–10% depending on the site measured) and not always sustained. The reason for a transient increase in bone

Table 7A Some drugs used in the treatment of osteoporosis

Inhibitors of bone turnover
Oestrogens
Progestogens
Tibolone
Calcitonins (salmon, eel, human)
Bisphosphonates
    Etidronate
    Clodronate
    Pamidronate
    Tiludronate
    Alendronate and others
Thiazide diuretics
Calcium
Vitamin D derivatives
    Calciferol and cholecalciferol
    Calcitriol
    Alfacalcidol
Ipriflavone

Stimulators of bone formation
Fluorides
    Sodium fluoride
    Monofluorophosphate
Anabolic steroids
    Stanozolol
    Oxandrolone
    Nandrolone
Parathyroid hormone and peptides
Intermittent calcitonin/phosphate
Ipriflavone

Transient state

mass is that the agents used to decrease bone turnover are generally inhibitors of bone resorption, which decrease the activation of new remodelling sites. Early during treatment, bone formation will continue at previously existing remodelling sites and bone mass will increase. Since bone turnover and its complete mineralization is a slow process, bone mineral mass may increase for several years before a new steady state is achieved (Parfitt, 1980). The duration of the transient response will also depend upon the abruptness and the degree with which an intervention inhibits activation so that if the long-term consequences of treatment are to be evaluated in patients with established osteoporosis, they must be studied for a period of at least 2 years and preferably longer (Kanis *et al*, 1991). Similarly, treatment-induced changes at 1 year cannot necessarily be expected to represent the changes which will occur thereafter.

Steady state

If the intervention used does not affect the balance between formation and resorption but only the rate of turnover, then bone loss will recur once the steady state has been attained, albeit with a lower rate of loss than before treatment. This predicted sequence of events, summarized in Figure 7.1 implies that the long-term effect of inhibitors of bone turnover is to decrease the rate of bone loss rather than to restore skeletal mass. The degree of effect is likely to differ depending on the prevailing rate of turnover at the time of intervention (see Fig. 7.1). There is some clinical evidence for this view, but it has been misinterpreted to imply that the responses in high-turnover osteoporosis are more complete. This is true of the transient increment in bone mass, but not necessarily for the steady-state responses.

The transient increments in bone mass are modest compared to the skeletal deficits encountered in patients with osteoporotic fractures. A conclusion might be that such agents are perhaps more suited to the prevention of bone loss rather than for restoring skeletal mass. However, a decrease in the rate of loss delays the time that an individual would reach a given value for bone density. Small changes in bone remodelling may induce long-term gains when viewed in this way since treatment will increase the time taken for an osteoporotic patient to reach a defined probability of fracture (Fig. 7.2).

This view of sequential changes in bone mass is an oversimplification.

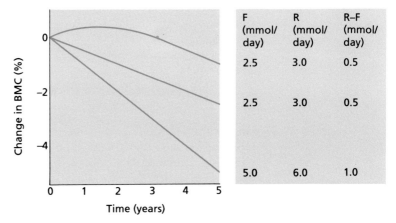

	F (mmol/ day)	R (mmol/ day)	R–F (mmol/ day)
	2.5	3.0	0.5
	2.5	3.0	0.5
	5.0	6.0	1.0

Fig. 7.1 Effects of altering bone turnover on bone mineral content (BMC) in osteoporosis. The relationship between BMC with time is shown for a patient losing 1% of bone mass per year due to an imbalance of bone at remodelling sites. In terms of calcium fluxes, more calcium is resorbed (R; 6 mmol/day) than formed (F; 5 mmol/day), a net deficit of 1 mmol/day representing a skeletal loss of 1% per annum. If bone turnover is halved without altering the imbalance between the amounts formed and resorbed then the rate of bone loss is halved. The administration of inhibitors of bone resorption permits, however, continued formation at pre-existing resorption sites so that BMC increases to infill this resorption space. When bone formation decreases to match the prevailing rate of bone resorption, bone loss will occur once more, but at a slower rate than before treatment.

Fig. 7.2 The effects of inhibiting bone turnover without affecting skeletal balance on rates of bone loss. (a) Shows the effects of placebo or calcium on rates of bone loss after oophorectomy and (b) the effects of oestrogens or placebo on bone loss after oophorectomy. In untreated patients a defined bone mass (and therefore fracture risk) is attained after 3–4 years whereas in the treated patients the attainment of the same risk is deferred. (Data based on Stepan *et al.*, 1989 and Lindsay *et al.*, 1976.)

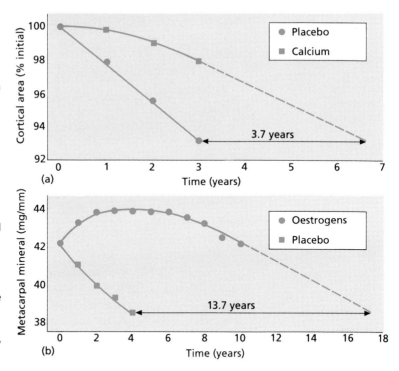

For example, under some conditions the bisphosphonates and calcitonin not only decrease bone turnover but also appear to decrease the depth of each resorption cavity. If the depth of erosion cavities is decreased, then the imbalance between resorption and formation, so characteristic of osteoporosis, may in fact be reversed, depending on the degree of this effect.

In addition, several agents alter the balance at remodelling sites by affecting the amount of bone formed within each erosion cavity. A good example is the anabolic steroids at endocortical sites. A component of the response to fluoride is also achieved in this way, at least in cancellous bone (see Chapter 8). Such effects, if persistent, would be expected to result in progressive gains of cancellous bone or cortical thickness.

In the long term, the rate of change in bone mass is directly related to the rate of activation of remodelling sites, whereas the direction of change depends upon the net balance between bone formation and resorption within remodelling units. Where the direction of change is positive, irrespective of the manner in which it is induced, bone mass should be increased rapidly if bone turnover can also be increased. This is the basis of ADFR or coherence regimes (Frost, 1969). The concept is one of **A**ctivating turnover to increase the rate of bone remodelling, thereafter to **D**epress with an inhibitor of bone resorption so that the depth of erosion cavities is decreased. There-

ADFR

Fig. 7.3 Schematic diagram to show remodelling imbalance at trabecular bone. (a) Shows imbalance at the remodelling site. If the depth of the erosion cavity is decreased sufficiently, the new bone formed over-corrects the imbalance (b). If activation frequency is increased, increments in bone density are induced more rapidly (c).

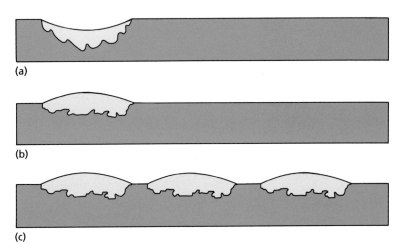

(a)

(b)

(c)

after, a **F**ree period is allowed so that a normal moiety of bone can form in a shallow erosion cavity and thereby increase skeletal mass. Finally, the process is **R**epeated (Fig. 7.3). There is some evidence that ADFR regimes might be more than a theoretical possibility and these are discussed subsequently.

A further way in which remodelling might be exploited is by disrupting the coupling process. As reviewed in Chapter 1, coupling is the phenomenon whereby osteoblasts are attracted to sites of previous resorption. Uncoupling is an important mechanism for bone loss, particularly in neoplastic bone disease. In this situation an erosion cavity fails to attract osteoblasts and progressive erosion may in time transect a trabecular structure or breach the cortex. Conversely, there can be positive uncoupling: the deposition of bone, not at sites of previous resorption, but at quiescent surfaces, or condensations of stromal elements within the marrow cavity to give rise to new bone formation. Both these changes are characteristic mechanisms for the induction of osteosclerotic metastases in which the normal trabecular architecture is overlaid by new bone deposited on quiescent surfaces. There is some indirect histological evidence that fluoride is capable of inducing new bone formation on previously quiescent bone surfaces (see Chapter 8).

The principles of bone remodelling in the cortex are essentially similar to those in cancellous bone (see Chapter 1).

As in the case of cancellous bone tissue, an increase in the activation frequency of bone remodelling (the birth rate of new remodelling units) will increase the resorption space and decrease the tissue mineral density. Conversely, a decrease in activation frequency will increase the apparent density but has perhaps less implications for structural strength. In contrast to cancellous bone, a resorption cavity cannot be overfilled due to

Coupling

Uncoupled formation

Cortical bone

These considerations suggest that apart from changes in the quality of bone, interventions to strengthen the skeleton at cortical sites will ultimately depend on thickening the cortex by endocortical or periosteal apposition of bone. Experimental agents, such as growth hormone and the prostaglandins, are capable of increasing periosteal apposition, and there is some evidence to suggest that endocortical apposition occurs with the use of anabolic steroids and prostaglandins.

EFFECTS ON QUALITY OF BONE

A potential concern with the use of inhibitors of bone turnover is that their major activity is to decrease the rate of bone remodelling. Whereas this may attenuate skeletal losses, it has been suggested that a very low rate of bone turnover might increase the risk of skeletal failure by reducing the rate of remodelling of fatigue-damaged

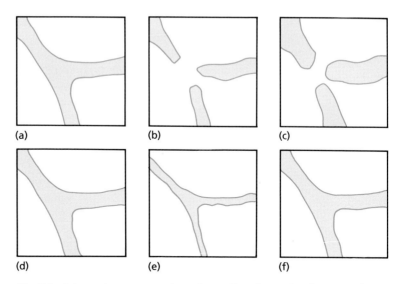

Fig. 7.4 Schematic representation of cancellous bone showing normal trabecular architecture and the thinning and discontinuity of trabecular elements (a–c). The disruption of continuity weakens the structure out of proportion to the amount of bone lost. Conversely, the deposition of new bone by influencing bone remodelling (c) may thicken remnant structures without necessarily restoring trabecular continuity. (d–f) Show trabecular thinning and the effect of a similar therapeutic intervention. (From Kanis, 1984.)

bone. Some support for this view comes from a study reporting spontaneous fractures in dogs treated with very high doses of clodronate. The doses used are likely to have inhibited bone turnover completely. However, states associated with less complete decreases in the rate of bone turnover are associated with lower incidence of fracture than higher turnover states. Furthermore, therapeutic suppression of bone turnover with oestrogen is associated with a decrease in fracture risk. Based on these considerations, it is likely that interventions which partially suppress turnover in postmenopausal women would not increase skeletal fragility. It is, nevertheless important that the long-term effects of interventions on turnover are examined as well as their effects on fracture.

A major limitation to the treatment of postmenopausal osteoporosis relates to the fact that all interventions currently being assessed exploit the remodelling process which is a surface-based event. When trabecular elements are lost the surface on which osteoblasts can be attracted by the coupling mechanism is destroyed (Fig. 7.4). Therapeutic manipulation of the remodelling process might be expected to thicken remnant structures without necessarily restoring trabecular continuity. On the other hand, a doubling in thickness of trabeculae increases its strength 10-fold. For these reasons the restoration of skeletal mass cannot necessarily be equated with the reversal of skeletal fragility. In corticosteroid osteoporosis, there is much less in the way of architectural abnormality. This suggests that the restoration of cancellous bone volume by the manipulation of bone remodelling is likely to restore mechanical competence of cancellous bone more completely in corticosteroid-induced osteoporosis than in hypogonadal states.

Agents which decrease the depth of resorption may have more marked effects on skeletal strength for any given change in bone mass, at least in cancellous bone. The average depth of erosion is approximately one-third of the trabecular width so that erosion itself may weaken a trabecula. A decrease in depth of erosion may therefore strengthen cancellous bone out of proportion to the amount gained.

Assessment of treatment on fracture

There are several problems to be taken into account in assessing the effects of intervention on vertebral fracture rates. Problems relate to the design of clinical trials and to the methodology used to assess fracture.

TRIAL DESIGN

The best way to improve a therapeutic outcome is to leave out the controls. Vertebral fracture is an episodic event and an event is

therefore followed by an event-free interval. Since patients usually come to medical attention at the time of an event, there will be an apparent decrease in fracture rates which may be mistaken for a treatment-induced effect (Kanis, 1984). Controls should be appropriately selected and historical controls not used. Indeed, the use of historical controls or those not randomly assigned may have contributed to the apparently beneficial effects of several agents. For this reason most would believe that evidence for efficacy should be based on prospective studies. The duration of exposure of controls should be the same as the duration of exposure in the test group where comparisons are to be made.

Problems with randomization

The most straightforward methodology is the double-blind randomized prospective study, but this is not without its own problems (Heaney, 1991). The objective of randomization is to improve the probability that the two (or more) groups are comparable so that treatment-induced effects can be confidently ascribed to the treatment. However, studies in osteoporosis are needed over relatively long time intervals, and drop-outs are to be expected (even in the most expert centres this may be as high as 15% per year). The assumptions made by the randomization at the start of the trial are unlikely to pertain at the point of comparison, namely the effects of treatment at 3 years. If drop-outs do not occur randomly but occur with greater frequency in a particular subgroup (e.g., patients with back pain think that the drug is not working) this will alter the apparent efficacy. An additional and more difficult problem to study is the effect of non-compliance which may differ between the treatment groups. Patients may take medicines more assiduously because of the development of pain or not take them because they do not think the medication is working.

ASSESSMENT OF FRACTURE

Problems in defining a fracture

Most fractures are clinically obvious but there are special problems in defining the presence or absence of vertebral fracture and the changes which occur in the natural history of the treated or untreated disorder. There is no gold standard for the definition of vertebral fracture. Small vertebral deformities occur with greater frequency than complete crush fractures and are commonly documented in trials of treatment because their frequency is higher. This in turn decreases the number of patients which is required for studies of efficacy. These fractures may, however, have less clinical significance than larger or symptomatic events. Thus, the more subtle the radiographic criteria used to diagnose fracture, the greater the risk that this is of no clinical significance (Kanis, 1984).

Definition of vertebral fracture

In judging the effects of intervention, many investigators have defined a new vertebral fracture as a decrease in vertebral height of between 15 and 25% in either the anterior, central or posterior height of the vertebral body. A fixed percentage decrease is not appropriate, however, since, for example, a 20% decrease in vertebral

Table 7.1 The effect of increasing false-positive rate on the apparent efficacy of a bone-active drug in a placebo-controlled trial. The true number of vertebral deformities is 60 in the placebo wing and the active agent has a true efficacy of 50, 33 or 20%. The apparent efficacy decreases as the false-positive rate increases. The bottom two rows show the effect of an uneven distribution of false-positive deformities. (From Kanis, 1993)

False-positive rate (%)*	Number of deformities in placebo wing	Apparent therapeutic efficacy (%)		
0	60	50	33	20
10†	65	45	30	18
20	75	40	27	16
30	86	35	23	14
40	100	30	20	12
50	120	25	17	10
60	150	20	13	8
70‡	200	15	10	6
70§	214	27	22	19
70‖	186	1	−4	−9

* Expressed as a percentage of the observed vertebral deformity rate.
† Rate as assessed by McCloskey *et al.* (1993).
‡ Rate as assessed by Melton *et al.* (1989).
§ 55% of false-positives in placebo wing.
‖ 55% of false-positives in active wing.

height can lie between 1 and 3 SD from the normal height depending on the vertebral level assessed and the site of the measurements (anterior, central or posterior) (McCloskey *et al.*, 1993). Thus many apparent deformities will be artefacts and many of the quantitative estimates used yield a very high false-positive rate.

This phenomenon clouds the interpretation of clinical trials in osteoporosis. A relatively high false-positive rate may decrease the apparent efficacy of an intervention when it is truly effective (Table 7.1). For example, in a double-blind prospective study of sodium fluoride (Riggs *et al.*, 1990) it was concluded that the frequency of vertebral fractures fell by 15%, which was not statistically significant. Given the known false-positive rate of the method used (70%), it is possible that the true effect was in the order of 33–50% (see Table 7.1), an effect more consistent with the earlier experience of the authors and others (see Chapter 8). Also, an unequal distribution of false-positive events will bias this estimate when the incidence of false-positives is high and the rate of real fractures is low. A practical example is provided in one of the studies examining the effects of etidronate on fracture frequency (Watts *et al.*, 1990). The rate of vertebral fracture fell from 63 to 30/1000 woman years in several hundred patients studied for 2 years. The rates are so low that the vast majority of apparent fractures are likely to be false-positives. We might postulate on this basis that, as luck would have it, a maldistribution of false-positives occurred in the test group. If so, longer follow-up periods would be likely to show a redistribution of false-positives. In other words, the effects should disappear, which is exactly what has been shown in the follow-up of this study.

There is currently general agreement that vertebral morphometry should be level specific, namely that algorithms should take into account the vertebral level. Most investigators would consider that only new vertebral events should be studied since the precision of measuring changes in previously deformed vertebrae is much less. In addition, the assignment of several criteria rather than a single criterion to judge fracture may improve the specificity without losing sensitivity. There are significant differences in vertebral height between communities so that appropriate normative references must be used. Many of these problems have only recently been identified so that many early studies of vertebral fracture rates are difficult to interpret.

Reference ranges

Calcium

Calcium is widely available throughout the world and is the major non-hormone replacement therapy (HRT) intervention used in osteoporosis. Whereas the role of calcium nutrition in the attainment of peak bone mass is controversial (see Chapter 2), there are now a substantial number of studies which indicate that calcium supplements (generally in excess of 1 g daily) are capable of slowing the rate of bone loss in women after the menopause with or without osteoporotic fractures. The evidence for this has been recently reviewed (Kanis, 1991) and several more recent publications support this view. Perhaps the most rigorous situation to test the effect of

Slows rate of bone loss

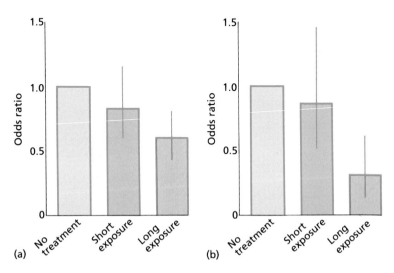

Fig. 7.5 Relative risk (±95% confidence intervals) of hip fracture in elderly women given (a) calcium supplements or (b) hormone replacement therapy. Both interventions showed a significant duration-dependent effect but the effects of calcium are less complete. (From Kanis et al., 1992.)

177 / Treatment with inhibitors of bone resorption

calcium is in women after oophorectomy, and placebo-controlled studies of the use of high doses of calcium suggest that the rate of bone loss may be halved, at least in cortical bone (see Fig. 7.2). Many other studies in women at or well after the menopause also show that pharmacological doses of calcium decrease the rate of cortical and cancellous bone loss.

> The effect of calcium in the treatment of osteoporosis appears to be due to its ability to decrease bone turnover.

It seems likely that this is related to the small increments in serum calcium and the resulting decrease in parathyroid hormone (PTH) and in the activation of bone turnover in much the same way as seen in younger individuals. Indirect evidence for such an effect is that calcium supplements are often associated with a small increase in skeletal mass and the induction of a transient state. The transient state may persist for up to 3 years at cortical sites (see Fig. 7.2). Similar but more rapid effects are observed at cancellous bone sites (Elders et al., 1991).

Until recently there were few adequate studies of the effect of calcium on fracture in women with osteoporosis. However, if bone loss can be delayed then it is reasonable to assume in this context that prevention of bone mass is an adequate surrogate for fracture frequency. A recent well-designed prospective study has shown that calcium supplements (1200 mg daily) decrease vertebral fracture frequency in women with established vertebral osteoporosis.

Some, but not all, epidemiological studies support the view that a high dietary intake of calcium decreases the risk of hip fracture (see Chapters 2 and 4). However, individuals who elect to take high calcium diets differ significantly from non-calcium-taking counterparts in terms of their general health, education and other possible confounding factors. But the risk of hip fractures also appears to be decreased in women taking pharmacological amounts of calcium

Table 7.2 Effects of calcium with vitamin D or placebo on the occurrence of extravertebral fractures in 3270 women. There was a significant decrease in femoral and other (non-vertebral) fractures ($P < 0.05$ and < 0.02, respectively). (From Chapuy et al., 1992)

Interval and follow up (months)	Treatment		Placebo	
	All fractures	Hip fractures	All fractures	Hip fractures
0–6	55	30	76	36
6–12	52	24	62	30
12–18	44	19	66	37
0–18	151	73	204	103

(Fig. 7.5). Of particular interest is that in one study calcium supplements were taken on average at the age of 70 years whereas the average age of hip fracture was 75 years. Thus treatment, even late in the natural history of bone loss, may have significant clinical dividends.

Calcium and vitamin D

In addition, a controlled prospective study in the elderly has shown that the use of calcium and vitamin D in the elderly significantly decreased the frequency of hip fracture. Over an 18-month follow-up 355 non-vertebral fractures occurred compared with 204 fractures in the placebo group. The decrease in both femoral and other non-vertebral fractures was significant (Table 7.2). It should be stated that these patients were drawn from a nursing home setting and some had coexisting vitamin D deficiency. Notwithstanding, the dose of vitamin D used was physiological and adds credibility to the less well-controlled studies suggesting that calcium with or without physiological doses of vitamin D decreases fracture risk. The prospective study also supports the view that the use of calcium and/or vitamin D, even relatively late in the natural history of osteoporotic bone loss, may have significant dividends in reducing the risk of hip fracture.

Effects in the elderly

This finding has obvious implications in devising treatment strategies for osteoporosis.

> It suggests that it is never too late to institute pharmacological programmes for the prevention of fracture.

If true, then this has many further implications. It may for example be appropriate to identify patients at risk at a much later age than is currently thought worthwhile. The later a long-term effective treatment is instituted, the greater the potential for cost-effectiveness.

WHO AND HOW TO TREAT

A wide variety of calcium preparations is available in most countries. Many non-proprietary forms are also available, but in many countries the calcium content is small, so that more than 10 tablets need to be taken daily in order to provide a dose of 1000 mg. There are small differences in the bioavailability of calcium between proprietary preparations but these are unlikely to be of therapeutic significance.

Achlorhydria

A possible exception is in patients with achlorhydria where calcium citrate is more efficiently absorbed, but this does not matter if calcium is taken with meals. Acute availability is greater with meals but again is of little therapeutic significance. It may be more important to divide the daily dose so that each dose does not exceed 500 mg or so since the gains from larger doses are trivial. It is important to recognize that the elemental content of calcium varies with the product. Calcium carbonate contains 40% of elemental calcium by weight, whereas calcium phosphate contains 31%, calcium lactate 13% and calcium gluconate 9%. In some non-proprietary brands the availability of calcium may be markedly reduced. The availability of calcium also varies in different foodstuffs, for example green vegetables, particularly spinach, appear to have significantly less than dairy products. Apart from this caveat, there is no reason to suggest that the consumption of calcium, particularly in the form of dairy products, would not have the same ultimate effect, though this has yet to be formally demonstrated.

In established osteoporosis, the risk of fracture is markedly increased following a first osteoporotic fracture. In such women it appears to be appropriate to offer an intervention and calcium is certainly a potential candidate. Some would go further and say that it is no longer ethical not to provide dietary calcium supplementation for patients with fractures. It is also reasonable to offer calcium either as a supplement or by dietary manipulation in all patients with osteoporosis in whom other treatments are not prescribed. It may also be reasonable to offer similar intervention to those in whom lifetime risk is unacceptably high. The major advantage of calcium is that it is easy to use, requires little monitoring and is acceptable to patients. Compliance with treatment is high (Elders et al., 1991). The major disadvantage is that the effects are less marked than with many other treatments.

SIDE EFFECTS
The risks of intervention with calcium or with physiological doses of vitamin D are negligible in otherwise healthy individuals (Elders et al., 1991). Side effects include bloating, flatulence and constipation but these are not common. Such agents should, however, not be given to patients with increased intestinal absorption of calcium such as hypercalciuric nephrolithiasis or sarcoidosis. For the same reason care should be exercised in patients taking vitamin D in pharmacological amounts or the 1α-hydroxylated derivatives. High intakes of calcium with alkalis may give rise to the milk-alkali syndrome but this is now a very rare occurrence.

The calcitonins

The physiological role of calcitonin in humans is uncertain. Though several disturbances in the secretion of calcitonin have been described in osteoporosis the relevance of such findings to treatment is insecure (see Chapter 3). Nevertheless, it is clear that calcitonin in pharmacological amounts is an inhibitor of bone resorption and this is a major reason for its use in osteoporosis.

PHARMACOLOGICAL PREPARATIONS
Several different calcitonins are available for the treatment of osteoporosis. Porcine calcitonin is extracted from pig thyroid glands, whereas the other calcitonins which are available are synthetic.

These include synthetic salmon (SCT; salcatonin), human (HCT) and a derivative of eel calcitonin (ECT).

Surprisingly, SCT resembles the human more than other mammalian calcitonins, and it is interesting to note that both SCT and ECT are more potent in humans than either the porcine or human hormone. In addition, SCT and ECT have a longer duration of hypocalcaemic activity.

EFFECTS ON BONE AND SERUM CALCIUM

Inhibits bone resorption
The major action of calcitonin is to inhibit bone resorption and thereby decrease plasma calcium and the urinary excretion of hydroxyproline. Since the pharmacological effect of calcitonin on bone is largely attributable to the number of functional osteoclasts, the degree of hypocalcaemia attained acutely after the injection of a fixed dose of calcitonin is proportional to the prevailing rate of bone resorption. The acute and medium-term responses are therefore greater in osteoporotic patients with higher rates of bone turnover as judged by scintigraphy or biochemical markers of disease activity.

Metabolic effects
It is to be expected that a decrease in serum calcium would provoke a homeostatic response. Secondary hyperparathyroidism occurs, but this is transient and matches the acute fall in serum calcium. Thus, repeated daily injections are associated with repeated but transient increases in PTH secretion. Repeated administration of calcitonin maintains the effect on resorption and is followed by a subsequent decrease in the serum activity of alkaline phosphatase. Histological findings after long-term treatment have shown decreases in both bone resorption and in bone formation (Gruber *et al.*, 1984) as expected of an inhibitor of bone resorption. This dissociation between the various aspects of bone remodelling is similar to that observed with the bisphosphonates (see p. 184).

Increased skeletal mass
During the early phase of treatment where bone resorption is inhibited but formation is still occurring at sites of previous bone resorption, it is to be expected that skeletal mass will increase. Traditional metabolic balance studies have shown an early increase in the calcium balance in patients with osteoporosis given parenteral calcitonin. More modern techniques have shown an increase in total body calcium as judged by neutron activation analysis or absorptiometric techniques (see below). The increase in skeletal mass does not continue indefinitely, but a new steady state is achieved when bone formation has been suppressed. Thus, increments in calcium balance become less marked with continued treatment. As expected, the new steady state of bone turnover takes many months to be achieved.

EFFECTS ON BONE MASS

Very little detailed dose-response work has been undertaken with the long-term use of parenteral calcitonin in osteoporosis, perhaps because of its safety, irrespective of the dose used. An early uncontrolled study in men and women with osteoporosis showed a variable response in total body calcium to 50–100 Medical Research Council units of synthetic SCT given three-times weekly with daily calcium supplements. More consistent effects were observed with 100 IU given daily which increased whole body calcium by 2% in the first year (Gruber *et al.*, 1984). Thereafter, increments in bone mass decreased and bone loss occurred at the end of the 26 months observation. Similar responses have been observed using absorptiometric techniques at many different sites with SCT or HCT. The dose most commonly used is 100 IU SCT daily, but lower doses of 50 IU are probably effective and in some studies have been given three-times weekly. The optimal dose regimen for prevention or treatment will probably now never be known since non-parenteral formulations have been developed which are likely to supplant the use of parenteral calcitonin.

Intranasal calcitonin has been more rigorously evaluated, both for prevention and treatment of osteoporosis. Thrice weekly regimens are probably ineffective. A randomized study over a 1-year period showed that bone loss at the spine could be prevented at the menopause over this period using 50 IU/day given by nasal spray for 5 days per week. The study is still in progress and to date bone loss appears to be prevented over a 5-year interval (Reginster, 1991). Similar results have been obtained in other studies over shorter periods (Overgaard *et al.*, 1989) on the lumbar spine, but 100 IU daily had little effect on total body mineral or forearm density, suggesting that larger doses might be required at cortical sites.

Nasally given calcitonin also prevents bone loss in osteoporotic patients (Thamsborg *et al.*, 1991). A regimen of 200 IU daily by nasal spray with calcium prevents bone loss at the forearm and the spine. Bone loss recurs when treatment is stopped so that some investigators have utilized an intermittent regimen (e.g., 1 year on, 1 off, 1 on). Over a 1- or 2-year period more marked effects on the lumbar spine are observed with 200 IU than with 50 or 100 IU given daily with calcium (Fig. 7.6). There were no measurable effects at the forearm, similar to effects noted in perimenopausal women. The optimal dose and treatment regimen is not established but bone loss appears to be attenuated for 5 years at the spine with intermittent exposure (year on/year off).

EFFECTS ON BONE PAIN

Several studies have been undertaken to determine whether the analgesic effect of calcitonin might be exploited in pain due to osteoporosis, particularly in the vertebral crush fracture syndrome. Controlled double-blind studies suggest an analgesic effect usually apparent 1 or 2 days after the start of treatment, as judged by the subjective evaluation of pain or the requirements for analgesics

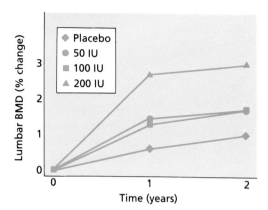

Fig. 7.6 Effects of different doses of nasal calcitonins given with calcium on bone mineral content (BMC) of the lumbar spine. (From Overgaard *et al.*, 1992.)

(Fig. 7.7). Regimens utilized have been HCT given parenterally three-times weekly, parenteral SCT and intranasally administered calcitonin. Effective doses of parenteral calcitonin appear to be about 100 IU daily of SCT, but analgesic responses, observed with 0.125 mg of HCT three-times weekly, suggest that even low doses may induce a substantial effect. The effects on bone pain as well as bone loss suggest a useful role for the acute management of fracture with calcitonin, particularly those in whom bed rest or other forms of immobilization are required.

EFFECTS ON FRACTURE

Vertebral and hip fracture

There are few data available on the effects of calcitonin on fracture rates. An open but randomized study has suggested a decrease in vertebral fracture frequency and more recently a prospective controlled study showed a decrease in vertebral deformities, but the number of events were few (Overgaard *et al.*, 1992). A retrospective survey in six European countries has shown an effect of calcitonin

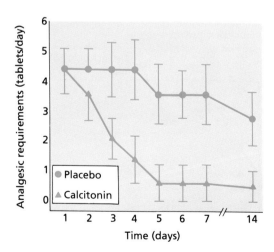

Fig. 7.7 The effects of subcutaneous salmon calcitonin (100 IU daily) or placebo given for 14 days on the requirements (mean ± SEM) for analgesics (paracetamol) in 56 patients. (From Lyritis *et al.*, 1991.)

with or without calcium on the risk of hip fracture after adjustment for potential confounding factors (Table 7.3).

SIDE EFFECTS

Nausea

When given parenterally all the calcitonins induce side effects which are inconvenient rather than serious. Nevertheless, they are a cause for stopping long-term treatment in 35% or so of patients. Their frequency and severity are dose dependent. The most frequent effect is nausea which occurs shortly after injection in up to 30% of patients. Nausea may be transient or persist for several hours. Occasionally, it may persist until the next injection and 5–10% of patients cannot tolerate long-term treatment for this reason. Nausea can be managed to some degree by the concurrent administration of antiemetics. Both can be given at bedtime.

Others

Other symptoms include flushing, vomiting, diarrhoea and local pain at the site of injection. The vascular effects are more marked in the young. Calcitonin appears to be remarkably safe and there are no known interactions of calcitonin with other drugs and no evidence of systemic toxicity to any organ.

Side effects are rarely, if ever, encountered with the use of nasal or rectal calcitonin. It is likely that this is related to the relatively low bioavailability of these formulations, and thus the lower dose of calcitonin delivered.

Bisphosphonates

The three bisphosphonates tested most widely are etidronate, clodronate and pamidronate. Over the past few years, many new bisphosphonates have become available for clinical testing (Fleisch, 1991) and several have been used in osteoporosis. In general there are more similarities than differences between bisphosphonates – at least in their ultimate therapeutic effect on bone – and they are for this reason reviewed collectively.

Table 7.3 Multivariate analysis of the effects of calcitonin and calcium on the risk of hip fracture. Note that the product of the odds ratio for the use of either agent alone (0.64) is similar to that for the combination suggesting an independent effect of each agent. (From Kanis et al., 1992)

Treatment combination		Relative risk	95% confidence interval	P
Calcitonin	Calcium			
No	No	1.00	—	—
No	Yes	0.82	0.63–1.07	0.149
Yes	No	0.78	0.48–1.27	0.318
Yes	Yes	0.63	0.44–0.90	0.012

CHEMISTRY, STRUCTURE AND
MECHANISM OF ACTION

General effects

The geminal bisphosphonates (also known as diphosphonates) are analogues of pyrophosphate (Fig. 7.8). The Pi-C-Pi structure accounts for its binding to bone mineral and its resistance to enzymatic hydrolysis. The major effects of the bisphosphonates on bone are to inhibit skeletal and extraskeletal calcification and to inhibit osteoclast-mediated bone resorption. They inhibit aortic, renal and dermal calcification induced by vitamin D. They also prevent periarticular calcification and articular changes associated with adjuvant arthritis. If given in high enough doses they inhibit the mineralization of bone and cartilage. This property led to the use of etidronate in heterotopic calcification following hip surgery or paraplegia. The inhibition of mineralization is thought to be due to the effects of bisphosphonate to inhibit crystal growth since there is a reasonably close relationship between the activities of different bisphosphonates on these systems (Shinoda et al., 1983).

Comparative potency

Whereas the effects of bisphosphonates on mineralization and crystal growth are in part dependent upon the Pi-C-Pi structure and its binding to hydroxyapatite, modifications of the side-chain appear to be important for the activity of bisphosphonates on bone resorption. For this reason, the activity of the different bisphosphonates on bone resorption varies markedly (a 10 000-fold range). The interest in the new bisphosphonates has been to develop compounds which dissociate the unwanted effects on mineralization from the effects on bone resorption.

Action on bone

Despite a large amount of experimental data, little is known of the way in which osteoclast-mediated bone resorption is affected by the bisphosphonates. The bisphosphonates are internalized by cells and rapid effects of bisphosphonates have been shown on the permeability of osteoclasts to calcium. Whereas direct effects of bisphosphonates have been shown on the ability of isolated osteoclasts to resorb bone, some studies show that the effects appear to be dependent on the prior adsorption of bisphosphonate onto bone. This suggests that a component of activity might depend on the presence of bisphosphonate on bone resorbing surfaces, rendering these unappetizing to the osteoclast.

Uptake in bone

Autoradiographic studies in experimental animals show the preferential localization of ^{3}H-alendronate at resorption surfaces (Sato et al., 1991). In the case of etidronate, similar studies suggest that localization occurs mainly at sites of bone formation, but probably relates to the much higher doses used. It seems likely that the mineral at resorption sites is readily saturated and that excess amounts are found at additional sites of accessible mineral such as at the mineralizing surface. The localization of bisphosphonates at resorption surfaces supports the view that bisphosphonate-laden bone is required to express their activity. Bound bisphosphonate can be

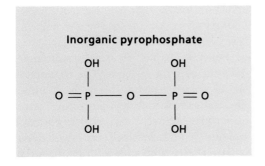

Inorganic pyrophosphate

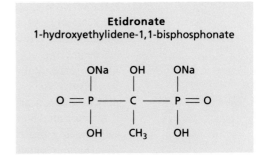

Etidronate
1-hydroxyethylidene-1,1-bisphosphonate

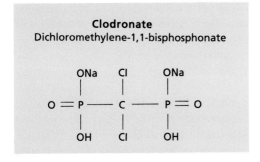

Clodronate
Dichloromethylene-1,1-bisphosphonate

Pamidronate
3 amino-1-hydroxypropylidene-1,
1-bisphosphonate

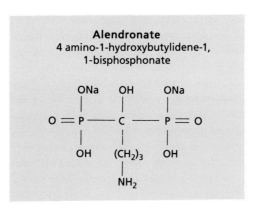

Alendronate
4 amino-1-hydroxybutylidene-1,
1-bisphosphonate

Neridronate
6 amino-1-hydroxyhexylidene-1,
1-bisphosphonate

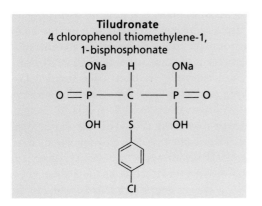

Tiludronate
4 chlorophenol thiomethylene-1,
1-bisphosphonate

Fig. 7.8 Structural formulae of pyrophosphate
and some of the bisphosphonates tested in
osteoporosis.

released from the bone surface by acidification and the acid micro-environment within the sealing zone of osteoclasts provides a mechanism for its release.

Decreased performance
of osteoclasts

Irrespective of the mechanism of action, the end result is to decrease the functional performance of osteoclasts. The results are likely to include a decreased depth of erosion cavities. The bisphosphonates also inhibit the development of osteoclast precursors to the multinucleate osteoclast cell pool. There are several possible consequences of such an activity. The first might be that fewer functional osteoclasts are available for recruitment to potential erosion sites, thereby decreasing the depth of the erosion cavity. A second is that the activation of new remodelling sites may be decreased. Both phenomena have been described in bisphosphonate-treated patients with osteoporosis.

PHARMACOLOGY AND KINETICS

Bisphosphonates are poorly absorbed from the gastrointestinal tract. Absorption is between 1 and 5% of the administered dose, but is reduced nearly to zero in the presence of calcium-containing foods or other divalent ions which chelate the bisphosphonate. Thus, the bisphosphonates, when given orally, need to be taken away from food or calcium-containing liquids.

Absorption

The half-life of all oral or injected bisphosphonates is short (20–120 minutes), in part related to rapid skeletal uptake. The initial volume of distribution approximates the extracellular fluid volume (approximately 25% body weight). None of the bisphosphonates currently tested have been shown to be metabolized and they are excreted unchanged almost exclusively in the urine. The renal clearance of bisphosphonates is approximately 50% of the glomerular filtration rate. However, there is significant protein binding of the bisphosphonates so that true renal clearance of free bisphosphonate may exceed the glomerular filtration rate, suggesting renal tubular secretion of the bisphosphonate. The amount of bisphosphonate appearing in the urine in normal subjects varies from 40 to 80%. The remainder is accounted for by skeletal retention.

Skeletal retention

The skeletal retention of bisphosphonates forms the basis of bone scanning and for using bisphosphonate retention to monitor bone metabolism. Skeletal retention of bisphosphonates is considerably increased in focal disorders such as Paget's disease and metastatic bone disease. The patchy distribution of bisphosphonates within the skeleton may have important therapeutic implications, since a proportionately greater dose of bisphosphonate is delivered to sites of disturbed skeletal metabolism than elsewhere. This targeting effect may have obvious pharmacological advantages in sparing non-affected sites, but may also cause problems in assessing the adequacy of a particular dose in focal causes of osteoporosis. Also, focal abnormalities such as fractures and microfractures also occur in generalized osteoporosis. The former are associated with increased bisphosphonate retention but the therapeutic relevance is not known.

Because bisphosphonates are incorporated into bone, and because the degree of skeletal uptake is dependent upon the prevailing rate of bone turnover, it is likely that the half-life of bisphosphonates is extremely long, perhaps several years, related to the turnover time of those skeletal sites. It has been suggested that the long skeletal half-life of bisphosphonate may account for the long duration of effect in postmenopausal osteoporosis. Relatively short exposures over days or weeks results in a prolonged decrease in bone resorption persisting for many months (Reginster *et al.*, 1989). This mechanism seems unlikely since in other disorders where increased bisphosphonate retention occurs (e.g., breast cancer metastatic to bone), the rate of reversal of therapeutic effect is relatively rapid after stopping treatment. For this reason, it seems likely that the skeletal retention of bisphosphonates in mineralized bone tissue is of little long-term clinical consequence.

Long skeletal half-life

EFFECTS ON SKELETAL METABOLISM

Extensive experience with the use of bisphosphonates in the treatment of osteoporosis has been obtained in many centres, but most studies have examined the effects on bone mass rather than on the more indirect indices of skeletal metabolism or on the histology of bone. A decrease in urinary hydroxyproline or other markers of bone resorption is an early effect of treatment and is followed by sequential changes in serum alkaline phosphatase.

Biochemical effects

During the early phase of such treatment it would be expected that the inhibition of bone resorption with continued bone formation, would decrease the net efflux of calcium from the skeleton to the extracellular fluid pool, lower serum calcium and the fasting urinary excretion of calcium and increase the secretion of PTH. This sequence of events has been described with pamidronate and clodronate in steroid-induced osteoporosis (Reid *et al.*, 1990) but incompletely with others. It is well described in Paget's disease where remodelling rates are higher and the effects of intervention more marked.

Different effect of etidronate

Similar effects have been inconsistently reported with low oral doses of etidronate (5–10 mg/kg daily) but they are not seen with higher doses. In osteoporosis, neither high oral (i.e., 20 mg/kg per day) nor high intravenous doses of etidronate decrease serum or urine calcium despite effective inhibition of bone resorption. This is due to the effect of etidronate to inhibit calcium accretion into bone concurrent with its action on bone resorption (McCloskey *et al.*, 1987). This adverse effect is minimized by its intermittent use. There is extensive evidence that the newer bisphosphonates do not impair the mineralization of bone even following high intravenous doses or after continuous oral treatment.

Histological studies indicate that all the bisphosphonates tested decrease the rate of turnover of bone. In addition, they may, under some circumstances, decrease the depth of erosion cavities which has been described with the use of intermittent etidronate, clodronate and continuous treatment with alendronate.

Skeletal architecture

The effects of the bisphosphonates on skeletal architecture have not yet been evaluated. It is likely, however, that any therapeutic manipulation of bone remodelling would thicken remnant trabecular structures without restoring trabecular continuity.

EFFECTS ON BONE MASS

The use of tiludronate, alendronate and pamidronate have been studied in the prevention of osteoporosis, the former in postmenopausal women and the latter in patients taking corticosteroids (Reid *et al.*, 1988; Reginster *et al.*, 1989). All these agents prevented bone loss over a year or two of observation. Clodronate has also been shown to prevent bone loss in postmenopausal and in several forms of secondary osteoporosis (see Chapter 9).

A number of bisphosphonates have been tested in patients with established osteoporosis. They include etidronate, clodronate, pamidronate, risedronate, tiludronate and alendronate. Several more are being evaluated in clinical studies. In general, they all appear to prevent further of bone loss.

Dose-response

Few dose-response studies have been undertaken, but where these have been done a dose-dependent effect is seen, at least in the rate of response (Fig. 7.9). Whereas many studies report an increase in skeletal mass, this is modest (2–10% depending on the site measured) and the early rate of increase has not been sustained as expected from the primary effect of the bisphosphonates to inhibit the activation of new remodelling sites. Thus, the increment is more in the first year than in the second year (Fig. 7.10). Few studies on bone mass have been conducted for sufficiently long periods to document the new steady state. An exception is a long-term study of the use of intermittent pamidronate, which shows changes in bone

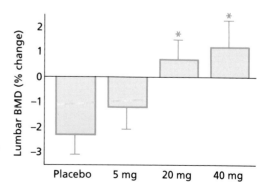

Fig. 7.9 Treatment-induced changes (% ± SEM) in the lumbar spine at 9 months following daily treatment with alendronate at the doses shown for 6 weeks. * Significantly different from placebo ($P<0.01$). BMD, bone mineral density. (From Harris *et al.*, 1993.)

189 / Treatment with inhibitors of bone resorption

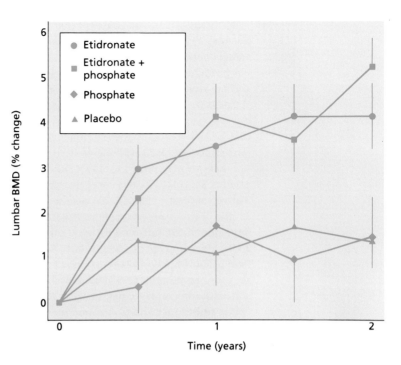

Fig. 7.10 Sequential changes in bone mineral density BMD; (mean ± SEM) of the lumbar spine following treatment with intermittent etidronate, phosphate, the combination of the two or placebo, all in conjunction with calcium. Note that the increment in bone density in the first year is substantially less than the increment in the second year. (From Watts *et al.*, 1990.)

Steady-state effects

mass at the forearm over several years which are consistent with the sequence of effects predicted from a decrease in bone remodelling (see Fig. 7.1). Similar effects have been observed with the intermittent use of clodronate (Fig. 7.11). Effects are seen at cortical and cancellous bone sites though, as expected, they are more marked at the latter and cortical sites did not increase significantly over baseline values.

In contrast, a study of the continuous administration of pamidronate (150 mg daily) showed an increase in bone mass which occurred

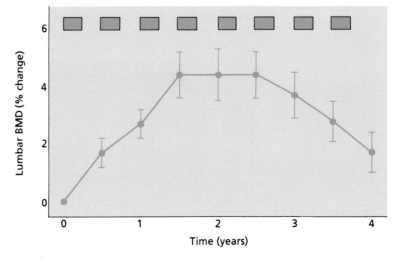

Fig. 7.11 Effects of intermittent clodronate by mouth (800 mg daily for 3 months out of 6) on lumbar bone mineral density (BMD; % change ±SEM). (Courtesy of C. Gennari.)

continuously for the duration of treatment. Results have been adequately shown over a 2-year treatment period, but less complete results suggest that this effect is sustained for up to 4 years (Table 7.4). However, a similar regimen in corticosteroid-induced osteoporosis has not shown progressive increments in bone mass at the forearm (see Chapter 9).

EFFECTS ON FRACTURE

The effects of bisphosphonates on fracture frequency in osteoporosis are not known with certainty. In the case of pamidronate, open studies suggest that vertebral fracture rates might decrease. Animal studies indicate that the compressive strength of bisphosphonate-treated vertebrae increases as expected for the changes induced in bone mass. Similar findings are noted for the bending strength of long bones suggesting that there is no impairment of the 'quality' of bone. Controlled studies with clodronate have shown a significant decrease in vertebral fracture frequency in patients with neoplasia affecting the skeleton (see Chapter 9).

The only controlled studies reported on fracture frequency in osteoporotic patients to date are with etidronate. Two randomized double-blind prospective studies report a decrease in vertebral fracture frequency (Storm *et al.*, 1990a,b; Watts *et al.*, 1990) with its intermittent use. In none of these studies was vertebral fracture a specified end-point and both have difficulties in interpretation. Both studies utilized criteria for vertebral fracture which are questionable. Moreover, the study from Denmark is on few patients (Storm *et al.*, 1990a) and the effects on fracture were not significant. Excluding the first year, the difference in fracture rates was significant over the subsequent 2 years. The sample size from the multicentre study in the United States is much greater (Watts *et al.*, 1990), but the incidence of new vertebral fractures is at first sight surprisingly low: eight- to 10-fold lower than in other studies examining vertebral osteoporosis so that the power is inadequate. One of the reasons for

Table 7.4 Changes in bone mineral content (BMC) at the lumbar spine in untreated patients with osteoporosis and patients given continuous treatment with pamidronate. (From Valkema *et al.*, 1989)

	n	BMC (rate of change; % per annum)
Untreated patients	19	0.4 ± 1.0
Treated patients	24	$3.1 \pm 1.0^*$
Excluding first year	23	$2.7 \pm 0.9^*$
Excluding first and second year	18	$3.7 \pm 1.1†$

* Significantly different from control values ($P < 0.05$).
† $P < 0.01$.

the low fracture rate may be that bone mineral density in this series of patients was not markedly reduced. Although the results of this study showed a decrease in vertebral fracture frequency the number of patients with fractures was low (6% of patients) and follow-up has shown that this trend was reversed. In reality, it may merely reflect a variable distribution of false-positive results.

BONE PAIN

Decreased bone pain

The bisphosphonates have been shown to decrease bone pain in a number of bone disorders. For example, pain relief has been observed in a number of double-blind studies in neoplastic bone disease affecting the skeleton (see Chapter 9). Relief of pain in the context of acute osteoporotic fractures has not yet been reported but is currently under study.

TREATMENT REGIMENS

At present etidronate is the most commonly used bisphosphonate and is widely licensed for use. Clodronate and alendronate are available for use in several countries. Many of the other bisphosphonates are in an advanced stage of clinical development and indeed several may become available in the near future. For this reason it may be useful to consider the regimens most frequently tested and likely used in clinical practice (Table 7.5).

Etidronate

Etidronate is used as a cyclical regimen since long-term continuous use adversely affects the mineralization of bone. Its intermittent use induces long-term suppression of bone turnover, but with minimal effects on bone mineralization. Four-hundred milligrams is given daily for 14 days every 3 months. In the interval, calcium 1250 mg is given daily. For obvious reasons it is important not to give etidronate continuously.

Etidronate is licensed for use in many countries for patients with established vertebral osteoporosis and there is currently no available evidence for a beneficial effect on other fractures. It is important that the agent not be given to patients with renal impairment since it may induce osteomalacia. It should also be avoided in patients with

Table 7.5 Treatment regimens shown to prevent bone loss in osteoporosis

Agent	Dose (mg)	Regimen	Comments
Etidronate	400	Two weeks out of 12	Given with calcium
Tiludronate	100	Daily	
Clodronate	800	Daily or daily every other month	
Pamidronate	150	Daily or intermittent	
Alendronate	5–20	Daily	

osteomalacia, and it may be prudent to stop treatment in the presence of appendicular fractures because it may impair fracture repair.

Clodronate

The dose of oral clodronate used in osteoporosis has ranged from 400 to 1600 mg daily, but the dose most widely used is 800 mg daily. As is the case for etidronate, it is evident that intermittent regimens can induce effects on skeletal metabolism for 1–2 years. The longer term effects on bone mass have not yet been well studied, but open studies suggest that clodronate behaves as expected of an inhibitor of bone turnover; namely a small increase in skeletal mass, followed by attenuated bone loss. It is not known whether continuous administration would induce more complete effects and this is the subject of current clinical studies.

Pamidronate

The most widely used regimen of pamidronate is 150 mg daily. It is the dose that has been shown to prevent glucocorticoid-induced bone loss over 2 years, and the regimen which has shown sustained effects on spinal bone mass over 4 years. Large-scale studies are now nearing completion in Europe which may provide further data on the long-term effects of continuous treatment.

Tiludronate

Alendronate

The optimal dose of tiludronate is not yet known. An oral dose of 100 mg daily for 6 months has been shown to prevent bone loss over 1 year (Reginster *et al.*, 1989). In the case of alendronate, the optimal dose appears to be 5–10 mg daily. These doses prevent bone loss in women shortly after the menopause as well as in patients with established osteoporosis.

SIDE EFFECTS

Very few side effects from treatment with bisphosphonates have been reported. The most frequently reported side effect is intestinal

Intestinal intolerance

intolerance, which occurs in about 10% of patients after oral treatment with etidronate or clodronate with doses of 800 mg daily or more. This can generally be avoided by splitting the daily dose. Pamidronate, also induces gastric intolerance in a minority of patients (10% or so) at the doses used in osteoporosis and may be a reason for stopping treatment. This may be a direct effect of high intraluminal concentrations of the amino derivatives since gastric effects of oral pamidronate are common where the dose requirements are higher. Lower doses of the more potent aminobisphosphonates, such as alendronate, may avoid this problem.

The rapid bolus injection of large amounts of bisphosphonates may precipitate acute renal failure, but this type of nephrotoxicity can be avoided by its slow intravenous infusion over 1 or 2 hours.

Etidronate

Etidronate appears to enhance renal tubular reabsorption of phosphate (TmP/GFR) which thereby increases serum phosphate. This effect is dose dependent and is generally seen with oral doses above 5 mg/kg per day. It is likely that hyperphosphataemia is not a unique feature of etidronate but is common to other bisphosphonates. The effect is of no known clinical significance.

Both intravenous and oral pamidronate induces a transient fever in 10–40% of patients. This effect is dose dependent, starts 24–48 hours after the onset of treatment and may persist for 1–2 days. Other changes include a transient decrease in peripheral lymphocytes and a decrease in serum zinc, consistent with an acute-phase response. The clinical significance of these changes or their relation to the mode of action of aminobisphosphonates is not known, but it is of interest that the response does not recur when patients are re-challenged. Infrequently reported side effects include rash, thrombocytopenia and an increase in bone pain. Similar effects are not observed with the more potent aminobisphosphonates such as alendronate at the dosage used in osteoporotic patients.

References

Chapuy MC, Arlot ME, DuBoef F *et al.* (1992) Vitamin D_3 and calcium to prevent hip fractures in elderly women. *N Engl J Med*; **327**: 1637–1642.

Elders PJM, Netelenbos JC, Lips P *et al.* (1991) Calcium supplementation reduces vertebral bone loss in perimenopausal women: a controlled trial in 248 women between 46 and 55 years of age. *J Clin Endocrinol Metab*; **73**: 533–540.

Fleisch H (1991) Bisphosphonates. *Drugs*; **42 (6)**: 919–944.

Frost HM (1969) Tetracycline based histological analysis of bone remodelling. *Calcif Tissue Res*; **3**: 211–237.

Gruber HE, Ivey JL, Baylink DJ *et al.* (1984) Long-term calcitonin therapy in postmenopausal osteomenopausal osteoporosis. *Metabolism*; **33**: 295–303.

Harris ST, Gertz BJ, Eyre DR, Genant HK, Survill TT, Chestnut CH (1993) The effect of short-term treatment with alendronate upon vertebral density and biochemical markers of bone remodeling in early postmenopausal women. *J Clin Endocrinol Metab*; **76**: 1399–1406.

Heaney RP (1991) How can we tell if a treatment works? Further thoughts on the randomized controlled trial. *Osteoporosis Int*; **1**: 215–217.

Kanis JA (1984) Treatment of osteoporotic fracture. *Lancet*; **i**: 27–33.

Kanis JA (1991) Calcium requirements for optimal skeletal health in women. *Calcif Tissue Int*; **49** (suppl.): 33–41.

Kanis JA (1993) What constitutes evidence for drug efficacy in osteoporosis. *Drugs and Aging*; **3**: 391–399.

Kanis JA, Geusens P, Christiansen C (1991) Guidelines for clinical trials in osteoporosis. *Osteoporosis Int*; **1**: 182–188.

Kanis JA, Johnell O, Gullberg B *et al.* (1992) Evidence for the efficacy of bone active drugs in the prevention of hip fracture. *BMJ*; **305**: 1124–1128.

Lindsay R, Hart DM, Aitken JM, McDonald EB, Anderson JB, Clarke AC (1976) Long term prevention of postmenopausal osteoporosis by oestrogen: evidence for an increased bone mass after delayed onset of oestrogen treatment. *Lancet*; **i**: 1038–1041.

Lyritis GP, Tsakalakos N, Magiasis B, Karachalios T, Viatzides A, Tsekoara M (1991) Analgesic effect of salmon calcitonin in osteoporotic vertebral fractures: a double-blind placebo-controlled clinical study. *Calcif Tissue Int*; **49**: 369–372.

McCloskey EV, Yates AJP, Beneton MNC *et al.* (1987) Comparative effects of intravenous diphosphonates on calcium and skeletal metabolism in man. *Bone*; **8** (suppl.): 35–41.

McCloskey EV, Spector T, Eyres KS *et al.* (1993) The assessment of vertebral deformity – a method for use in population studies and clinical trials. *Osteoporosis Int*; **3**: 138–147.

Melton LJ, Kan SH, Frge MA, Wahner HW, O'Fallom WM, Riggs BL (1989) Epidemiology of vertebral fractures in women. *Am J Epidemiol*; **129**: 1000–1011.

Overgaard K, Riis BJ, Christiansen C, Hansen MA (1989) Effect of salcatonin given intranasally on early postmenopausal bone loss. *Br Med J*; **299**: 477–479.

Overgaard KY, Hansen MA, Jensen SB, Christiansen C (1992) Effect of salcatonin given intranasally on bone mass and fracture rates in established osteoporosis: a dose-response study. *BMJ*; **305**: 556–561.

Parfitt AM (1980) Morphological basis of bone mineral measurements: transient and steady state effects of treatment in osteoporosis. *Miner Electrolyte Metab*; **4**: 273–287.

Reginster JY (1991) Effect of calcitonin on bone mass and fracture rates. *Am J Med*; **91** (suppl. 5B): 19–22.

Reginster JY, Lecart MP, Deroisy R *et al.* (1989) Prevention of postmenopausal bone loss by tiludronate. *Lancet*; **ii**: 1469–1471.

Reid IR, King AR, Alexander CJ, Ibbertson HK (1988) Prevention of steroid-induced osteoporosis with (3-amino-1-hydroxypropylidene)-1,1-bisphosphonate (APD). *Lancet*; **i**: 143–146.

Reid IR, Schooler BA, Stewart AW (1990) Prevention of glucocorticoid-induced osteoporosis. *J Bone Miner Res*; **5**: 619–623.

Riggs BL, Hodgson SF, O'Fallon WM *et al.* (1990) Effect of fluoride treatment on the fracture rate in postmenopausal women with osteoporosis. *N Engl J Med*; **22**: 802–809.

Sato M, Grasser W, Endo N *et al.* (1991) Bisphosphonate action: alendronate localization in rat bone and effects on osteoclast ultrastructure. *J Clin Invest*; **88**: 2095–2105.

Shinoda H, Adamek G, Felix R *et al.* (1983) Structure–activity relationship of various bisphosphonates. *Calcif Tissue Int*; **35**: 87–99.

Stepan JJ, Pospichal J, Presl J, Pacovsky V (1989) Prospective trial of ossein-hydroxyapatite compound in surgically induced postmenopausal women. *Bone*; **10**; 179–185.

Storm T, Thamsborg G, Steiniche T *et al.* (1990a) Effect of intermittent cyclical etidronate therapy on bone mass and fracture rate in postmenopausal osteoporosis. *N Engl J Med*; **322**: 1265–1271.

Storm T, Thamsborg G, Steiniche T *et al.* (1990b) Etidronate for postmenopausal osteoporosis. *N Engl J Med*; **323**: 1209–1210.

Thamsborg G, Storm TL, Sykulski R *et al.* (1991) Effect of different doses of nasal salmon calcitonin on bone mass. *Calcif Tissue Int*; **48**: 302–307.

Valkema RF, Vismans JFE, Papapoulos SE *et al.* (1989) Maintained improvement in calcium balance and bone mineral content in patients with osteoporosis treated with the bisphosphonate APD. *Bone Miner*; **5**: 183–192.

Watts NB, Harris ST, Genant HK *et al.* (1990) Intermittent cyclical etidronate treatment of postmenopausal osteoporosis. *N Engl J Med*; **323**: 73–79.

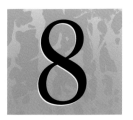

Other agents for generalized osteoporosis

8

Although there is much to be learned about the inhibitors of bone resorption, they all more or less decrease the activation frequency of bone. A number of other agents are used or are being developed for the treatment of osteoporosis (see Table 7 A) but their effects on bone or on other target tissues are more complex and are described below.

Fluorides

Efficacy of fluoride controversial

Fluoride is a trace element present in all human tissue. It has a particular affinity for bone tissue and accumulates in other tissues in which calcification occurs. It has been used for more than 30 years in the management of osteoporosis and is one of the few agents which has marked anabolic effects on the skeleton. The efficacy of fluoride regimens continues, however, to be the subject of considerable controversy. One of the problems is its 'age' and much of the early work undertaken utilized methodology and outcomes which are unacceptable today. A further problem is that sodium fluoride as a treatment is cheap and not patented (though some formulations are), so that it has been difficult for investigators or industry to make the investments required to undertake a modern programme of evaluation.

PHARMACOKINETICS

Preparations of fluoride include sodium fluoride as a tablet and enteric-coated or sustained-release preparations. Disodium mono-fluorophosphate (Na_2PO_4F) is available in many European countries. A dose of 200 mg is equivalent to 16.4 mg of fluoride ion (or 36 mg sodium fluoride). The absorption of fluoride salts is rapid and maximal serum concentrations are seen after half an hour and is cleared rapidly from the circulation.

Absorption

The absorption of sodium fluoride solution is near 100% and occurs by simple diffusion through the gastrointestinal wall. In the small intestine with a higher pH, fluoride is in its anionic form and is able to form salts less soluble than sodium fluoride. For these reasons the use of sustained-release or enteric-coated formulations decreases the bioavailability and there is a greater variability in absorption than that observed with sodium fluoride solutions. With the exception of monofluorophosphate salts, bioavailability is significantly reduced with food and in the presence of calcium or antacids so that calcium salts, commonly given in treatment regimens with fluoride should be taken separately. Apart from the dose delivered, alterations in the pharmacokinetic profile of delayed- or sustained-release preparations are unlikely to have any skeletal significance, since it is the total cumulative dose delivered to the skeleton which is of importance. The advantage of delayed-release preparations lies principally in their fewer side effects.

The non-renal clearance of fluoride (approx 80 ml/minute) mainly reflects accretion into bone (Ekstrand *et al.*, 1978). The uptake of fluoride by bone is not homogeneous and proportionately more is taken up by cancellous than by cortical bone. Thus, in osteoporotic and healthy individuals the skeletal uptake of fluoride will differ, and within each patient is not uniform. The patchy distribution of fluoride within the skeleton may have therapeutic implications since proportionately greater doses are delivered to sites with greater metabolic activity or vascular supply. This may account to some extent for the heterogeneity of response observed in clinical studies and for the induction of stress fractures.

Skeletal uptake

PHARMACOLOGY

Effects on bone mineral

Fluoride decelerates the conversion of amorphous calcium phosphate to octacalcium phosphate, but also promotes the hydrolysis of octacalcium phosphate to hydroxyapatite. The integrated effect is to promote the production of hydroxyapatite and this may be a physiological effect of fluoride (Merz, 1981). At pharmacological concentrations, fluoride promotes the development of a more stable bone apatite. Bone apatite contains less hydroxyl ions than hydroxyapatite resulting in open spaces which decrease the stability of the apatite lattice. Since the fluoride ion has about the same size and shape as the hydroxyl ion it can readily substitute isomorphically. Both fluorapatite and fluor-hydroxyapatite are less soluble than hydroxyapatite which may render bone more resistant to osteoclast-mediated bone resorption.

More stable bone apatite

Dose-dependent effects

Moderate fluoride exposure is associated with an increase in width of hydroxyapatite crystals, but fluorosis is associated with an increase in length of crystal structures, possibly associated with the non-lamellar (woven) deposition of bone matrix. Thus, 'physiological' quantities of fluoride (less than 2 mg daily) appear to promote hydroxyapatite formation, therapeutic quantities promote the production of fluor-apatite increasing the stability of the mineral phase, and toxic amounts of fluoride (fluorosis) radically alter crystal morphology.

'Physiologic' doses of fluoride decrease the incidence of dental caries in childhood but have no demonstrable effect on bone structure. Under steady-state conditions the bone fluoride concentration is less than 2500 ppm. An intake of 2–4 mg daily will induce mottling of enamel of erupting teeth without demonstrable effects on bone (2500–5000 ppm). An intake of 8 mg daily produces a 10% incidence of radiographically apparent osteosclerosis. Endemic and industrial fluorosis is evident when humans are exposed to 25–80 mg/day for 10–20 years with bone fluoride values greater than 0.5%.

Effects on collagen formation and mineralization

Effect on osteoblasts

At therapeutic concentrations fluoride has been shown to increase the proliferation of osteoblast-like cells *in vitro*, suggesting a direct mitogenic effect (Farley *et al.*, 1983). Although high doses of fluoride are associated with increased numbers of osteoblasts, they appear less plump than normal (Kanis & Meunier, 1984). In addition, doses of fluoride (>20 mg daily, equivalent to 44.2 mg sodium fluoride or higher) increase the time interval between the onset of matrix formation and its subsequent mineralization (Eriksen *et al.*, 1985). Even higher doses of fluoride induce woven rather than lamellar bone formation and obvious osteomalacia (Baylink & Bernstein, 1967). These effects are dose dependent and are modified by high intakes of calcium or by vitamin D.

Dose dependency and the effects of calcium

Fluorosis is characterized by dense osteosclerosis, and also by exostoses, ligamentous calcification, neurological complications due to bony overgrowth and osteoarthritis. These manifestations are associated with osteomalacia and woven bone formation.

Fluorosis

Early experience with the use of sodium fluoride for the treatment of osteoporosis reproduced some of the features of fluorosis. Subsequent studies with variable doses of sodium fluoride with vitamin D (50 000 IU twice weekly) indicated that lower doses (60–90 mg daily) were capable of stimulating bone formation and that the addition of calcium supplements (>900 mg daily) abolished the increase in bone resorption surfaces seen with the use of fluoride and vitamin D alone and decreased the formation of excessive unmineralized osteoid.

Vitamin D

The addition of vitamin D is associated with an appreciable incidence of vitamin D toxicity, but in other respects, the clinical outcome is similar to that in patients treated with fluoride and calcium supplements alone (Riggs *et al.*, 1982). This suggests that doses of fluoride in excess of 20 mg daily might be given with calcium supplements alone in order to avoid defective mineralization of bone and secondary hyperparathyroidism. High doses of vitamin D are likely to accelerate cortical losses.

Biochemical effects

The biochemical effects of fluoride alone are difficult to assess since most treatments have used calcium and/or vitamin D. Most investigators report little or no change in plasma or urine calcium and phosphate values with long-term treatment. Hypercalciuria and hypercalcaemia are attributable to vitamin D toxicity (Riggs *et al.*, 1982). The effects of fluoride on parathyroid hormone (PTH) secretion appear to depend upon changes in serum calcium. Thus, marked secondary hyperparathyroidism occurs in endemic fluorosis, when associated with poor nutrition for calcium and vitamin D. Little change is observed in clinical use when given with calcium supplements (Riggs *et al.*, 1990).

Sodium fluoride induces the expected changes in indirect indices of skeletal metabolism. Plasma activity of alkaline phosphatase and osteocalcin commonly increase, consistent with the stimulation of osteoblast numbers.

Effects on bone remodelling

Detailed histomorphometric studies in humans have examined the effects of sodium fluoride (40–60 mg/day) given for 5 years in women with spinal crush fracture (Eriksen *et al.*, 1985). Patients were also treated with calcium (45 mmol/day) and calciferol 18 000 IU/day. Cancellous bone volume increased markedly. The depth of resorption cavities does not increase, but the mean thickness of new bone structural units is increased. Woven bone formation did not occur at this dose indicating that increases in the volume of bone formed are not due to the higher volume occupied by woven bone. The time to complete a remodelling sequence in fluoride-treated patients is prolonged from 1 to 3 years. All phases of remodelling (resorption, formation and mineralization) are affected. This suggests that the increases observed at the resorption surface are not solely due to increased bone resorption but to a longer but less efficient period of resorption at each remodelling site (Fig. 8.1). There is also some evidence that fluoride induces uncoupled bone formation.

Because the time to form or resorb a moiety of bone is increased, the surfaces of bone occupied by formation are also increased. This should not be misinterpreted to denote osteomalacia.

There have been relatively few studies concerning the effects of sodium fluoride on the architecture of cancellous bone. In our own studies the restoration of skeletal mass was associated with substantial thickening of trabecular elements, but with no increase in their connectivity (Aaron *et al.*, 1991).

CLINICAL EFFECTS

Radiographic effects

Many uncontrolled studies have described increases in bone density

---

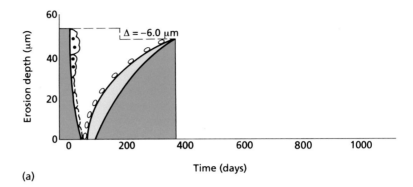

(a)

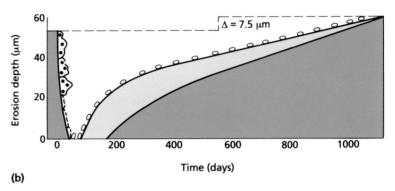

(b)

Fig. 8.1 Schematic reconstruction of remodelling event on the surface of trabecular bone (a) before and (b) after treatment with sodium fluoride. (a) Shows the average time to complete erosion and formation. The y-axis shows the depth of erosion and in the untreated patient the inadequate formation results in a net deficit of 6 μm in wall thickness. (b) During treatment all aspects of remodelling are prolonged. An increase in osteoid width is due to the delay between the onset of matrix formation and its mineralization. The depth of erosion is normal but treatment results in a net gain in bone mass since erosion cavities are overfilled by 7.5 μm. The treatment induced an increase in wall thickness (13.5 μm) representing a 30% increase over pretreatment values (From Eriksen *et al.*, 1985.)

Increased trabecular markings

in the axial skeleton. These changes include coarsening and increased prominence of trabecular markings and thickening of the vertebral end-plates. Radiographic improvement has been noted in 30–60% of patients given long-term treatment.

Effects on bone mass
Effects on cancellous bone at the spine are dramatic (Fig. 8.2). Indeed, vertebral bone mineral mass may increase in osteoporotic patients to values within the normal range within 5 years. Cancellous bone of the appendicular skeleton is responsive to fluoride.

Variable response

Up to 40% of patients show little or no improvement in bone mass (Briancon & Meunier, 1981; Harrison *et al.*, 1981). The reasons for

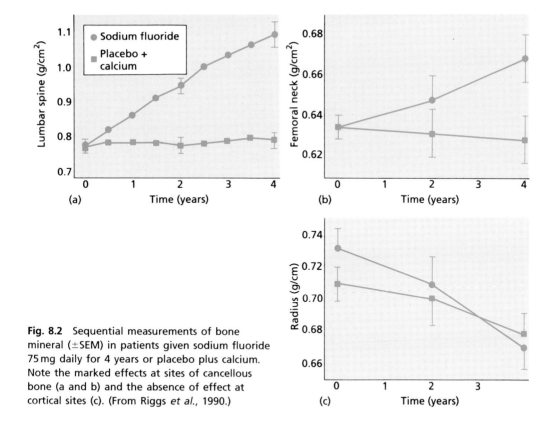

Fig. 8.2 Sequential measurements of bone mineral (±SEM) in patients given sodium fluoride 75 mg daily for 4 years or placebo plus calcium. Note the marked effects at sites of cancellous bone (a and b) and the absence of effect at cortical sites (c). (From Riggs *et al.*, 1990.)

Less effect on cortical sites

this variability are not known. The anabolic actions on cancellous bone are not associated with comparable effects at cortical sites. Indeed studies have not shown changes in bone density at the cortical sites of the forearm (see Fig. 8.2). When high doses are used without calcium, a decrease in metacarpal and femoral cortical width occurs (Dambacher *et al.*, 1978). This is most likely related to an increase in PTH secretion.

Effects on bone strength and fracture

Experimental studies suggest that fluorotic bone is more resistant to compressive forces, but more easily fractured by torsional strain. The effect of fluoride on bone strength is bimodal. Modest doses increase strength in experimental animals and high doses or continued exposure decrease strength. Thus, the ultimate arbiter of efficacy is the effect of treatment on fracture.

Decrease in vertebral fractures

Many studies show a decrease in vertebral fracture frequency in patients treated with sodium fluoride, but the majority have been poorly controlled. Several of these studies have reported that the effects of fluoride on fracture frequency depend upon the increment in bone mass induced by treatment as judged by densitometry or radiographic changes (Table 8.1). Although the analyses are retrospective, the differences in risk are striking.

A more adequately controlled, but open study evaluated the effects of sodium fluoride 50 mg daily (with calcium and vitamin D) and compared these with a variety of other commonly used treatments. Over a 2-year treatment period, the fluoride-treated patients showed a significantly lower rate of new vertebral fractures (Mamelle *et al.*, 1988). A more recent but unpublished randomized study showed that 50 mg daily of sodium fluoride significantly decreased the vertebral fracture rate (Buckle, 1989).

Restoration of bone mass

In contrast, two recent double-blind prospective studies from the United States have shown no significant effect of sodium fluoride on vertebral fracture frequency (Kleerekoper *et al.*, 1990; Riggs *et al.*, 1994). In the largest of these, 202 patients were given 90 and 60 mg of sodium fluoride on alternate days with 1500 mg of calcium. Bone mineral density (BMD) at the lumbar spine increased by 34% in the 135 patients evaluated at 4 years (see Fig. 8.2). The decrease in vertebral fracture rate was 15% and was not statistically significant. The other study showed no effect of fluoride on the fracture rate.

Dose-dependent effects

A variety of opinions have been offered to explain the apparent difference in outcome between the American and European studies. These may relate to the doses of sodium fluoride used. In the North American studies the dose utilized (75 mg/day) was substantially higher than the doses commonly used in Europe. Moreover, the bioavailability of formulations utilized in Europe is lower, so that the daily dose was 2½-times greater than that used in other studies demonstrating significant effects on vertebral fracture frequency (Table 8.2). Such doses induce osteomalacia in some patients. In a further analysis of their data, those patients treated with more modest doses of fluoride (< 60 mg daily) fared significantly better in terms of fracture rates.

A second reason for the discrepancy may relate to the method of the assessment of vertebral fracture rates. The algorithm used has

Table 8.1 Comparison between patients according to the effects of fluoride on bone mineral density (BMD). (From Farley *et al.*, 1992)

	Non-responders	Responders*
Number of patients	131	258
Dose of fluoride (mg/d)†	28 ± 8	31 ± 7
Time on fluoride (months)†	18 ± 15	28 ± 17
Initial BMD (mg/ml)‡	64 ± 32	62 ± 28
Fracture rate/100 patient years†	12	5

* A response defined as an increase in lumbar BMD of more than 8 mg/ml by quantitative computed tomography.
† $P < 0.001$.
‡ $P =$ NS.

Table 8.2 Differences between therapeutic regimens of sodium fluoride in the treatment of established vertebral osteoporosis. (Data from Nagant de Deuxchaisnes et al., 1990)

	Riggs et al. (1990)	Mamelle et al. (1988)	Difference (%)
Dose used (mg/day)	75	50	+50
Bioavailability	85	53	+60
Duration of treatment (years)	4	2	+100
Total exposure (g)	93	19	+389

very high false-positive rates which decreases the apparent effect of intervention (see Chapter 7).

Symptoms

Backpain

Many studies report symptomatic relief of backache, but these reports come from uncontrolled trials. One randomized clinical trial showed relief of backache after 3 months of treatment with the combination of fluoride, vitamin D and calcium compared to placebo.

Adverse effects

Side effects common

Side effects of fluoride therapy are common, but mainly transient. They include gastrointestinal irritation (nausea, vomiting, pain, diarrhoea and occasionally gastrointestinal bleeding) and arthralgic, bony, or periarthralgic pain. In a review of the literature, treatment was estimated to have been stopped because of side effects in 30 of 350 cases (8%) (Briancon & Meunier, 1979). The side effects of fluoride and their frequency depend on the dose, its formulation and the time of administration. Gastrointestinal side effects appear to be most troublesome with solutions and are improved by tablet formulations and when taken with food (Parsons et al., 1983). Fewer gastrointestinal side effects are noted with sustained release or enteric coated preparations.

Osteoarticular pain

Osteoarticular pain is the other major side effect of sodium fluoride. Its incidence is also dose dependent and it commonly resolves after stopping treatment over 4–8 weeks. It has now become apparent that limb pain associated with fluoride treatment may sometimes be due to the presence of microfractures visible on bone scans. Occasionally, incomplete fissure fractures have been noted which are evident on X-ray once callus formation has occurred (Fig. 8.3; Schnitzler,

Microfracture

1984) These fractures occur most commonly in patients with the lower BMD. In some, pain may herald complete fractures and pain is a reason for withdrawing treatment. Treatment may be resumed at a lower dose when bone pain has ceased. The phenomenon may be caused by the high fluoride uptake at the site of microfractures which are common in osteoporosis. High focal concentrations are likely to inhibit their repair.

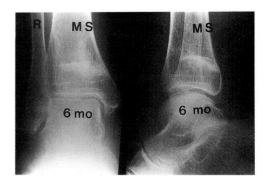

Fig. 8.3 Radiograph to show the presence of a callus at the distal tibia in a patient given sodium fluoride several weeks after the onset of bone pain.

Increased risk of hip fracture?

For this reason there has been concern that the incidence of hip fracture may be increased in patients given fluoride. In a large randomized series of elderly women, the administration of 50 mg daily of sodium fluoride for 6 months resulted in an increase in the fracture rate compared to placebo, but no calcium supplements were given. Because of this concern, Riggs *et al.* (1987) combined the retrospective data from five medical centres. The incidence of hip fracture was similar to that observed before treatment suggesting that fluoride did not increase this risk. The choice of centres was clearly biased, and in the controlled prospective study from Rochester, the large doses used were associated with a significant increase in the risk of non-vertebral fractures (relative risk 1.9; 95% confidence intervals, 1.1–3.4). Eight fractures of the proximal femur occurred in the fluoride-treated group and three in the calcium-treated controls.

Not all studies have shown an increase in appendicular fractures. Where calcium and vitamin D were prescribed concurrently, a 2-year controlled study in 180 osteoporotic patients showed no increase in hip or long-bone fractures (Mamelle *et al.*, 1988). Vose *et al.* (1978) undertook a long-term follow-up of males treated with fluoride, and found fewer hip fractures in fluoride-treated patients compared to those given oxymethalone or placebo.

CLINICAL USE
The balance of probabilities is that fluoride significantly decreases the risk of vertebral fracture. Well-designed trials with appropriate doses and appropriate methods of evaluating fractures are needed to determine this beyond a reasonable doubt. In the clinical use of fluoride, it would seem prudent to avoid its use in patients with marked cortical osteoporosis because of the risk of hip fracture. In Choice of dose order to minimize the risk of hip fractures the dose chosen should be appropriate taking into account the bioavailability of the preparation. A reasonable regimen would be to supply 15–25 mg fluoride ion daily.

The use of sodium fluoride at the recommended doses is associated with a significant incidence of side effects which are reversed when treatment is stopped. Enteric-coated preparations cause fewer gastro-intestinal side effects than a sodium fluoride solution or tablets. Other side effects, particularly the arthralgic and periarthralgic side effects also appear to be dose dependent. All these side effects can be of clinical significance, and up to 10% of patients cannot tolerate treatment.

There is no clearly definable consensus on how to monitor treatment. Many centres with an interest in the disorder monitor serum and urine fluoride levels, but these are not widely available and add an extra complexity of doubtful value to management.

Monitoring response

A major problem in management is that the response to treatment is heterogeneous and up to 40% of patients show little or no anabolic effect of sodium fluoride. There is currently no reliable way of assessing before treatment who will respond poorly or favourably. There is some evidence to suggest that those patients in whom no change in serum activity of alkaline phosphatase is observed also show no increase in trabecular bone mass. Marked increases in phosphatase may also, however, herald osteoarticular symptoms and may be a reason for decreasing the dose. Effects on bone mass can be assessed either by assessment of BMD or by radiographic assessment of the spine.

Relative contraindication

Fluoride should be used cautiously in patients with renal failure and in such patients serum fluoride measurements are likely to be of value. In the elderly, the presence of osteomalacia should be excluded before treatment is started since patients are likely to respond adversely to fluoride unless vitamin D is also given. This suggests that physiological doses of vitamin D should be given where the nutritional status of patients is in doubt, but pharmacological doses of vitamin D offer no advantages over the use of fluoride and calcium alone. The use of calcium supplements (1 g or more daily) minimizes unwanted effects on mineralization and decreases the fluoride-induced resorption of bone.

It is unclear for how long treatment should be given. There appears to be good evidence from the literature on fluorosis that doses should not be continued indefinitely. It seems reasonable to attempt to restore skeletal mass to within the normal range, which in most patients can be achieved within 5 years. Bone loss recurs when treatment is stopped so that retreatment several years later may be required.

Testosterone and the anabolic steroids

The potential use of androgens and anabolic steroids for the treatment of osteoporosis has been appreciated since the early 1940s. The early studies of calcium balance showed that a markedly positive skeletal balance could be induced by treatment with testosterone, either alone or in combination with oestrogen therapy. However, osteoporosis is predominantly a female problem and the masculinizing effects of androgens in women made these agents unacceptable as a treatment for postmenopausal osteoporosis.

Anabolic index

Over the last 25 years many synthetic anabolic steroids have been available for therapeutic use which are analogues of testosterone but which have fewer androgenic effects. The term anabolic describes the relative androgenic effects compared to the effects on muscle mass. The anabolic index refers to the relative activity of these compounds on the hypertrophy of the levator ani muscles of the castrated rat compared to their effects on the seminal vesicles. The ratio of anabolic to androgenic effect of compounds used varies markedly but is dose dependent.

Types of agent

Anabolic steroids can be broadly divided according to structural additions at the carbon 17 position. 17-α-alkylalated agents include stanozolol and oxymethalone. 17-β-esterified derivatives include testosterone and nandrolone. The side effect profile is determined in part by these different conformations. In addition, a variety of additional structural diversity is found including additional ring structures adjacent to the A ring. Examples include stanozolol and danazol (used for endometriosis).

Anabolic steroids most commonly used in osteoporosis are stanozolol and nandrolone but they are not universally approved for use. Stanozolol is given by mouth. The most common route for nandrolone is by intramuscular injection of nandrolone decanoate. It is given as a depot injection which increases its half-life to approximately 6 days. Other agents tested in osteoporosis are danazol, oxymethalone, oxandrolone and methandrostenolone. Tibolone has weak androgenic, progestational and estrogenic activity. Its use in osteoporosis is described in Chapter 6.

BIOCHEMICAL EFFECTS

Decreased urinary excretion of calcium

The biochemical changes induced by anabolic steroids in postmenopausal women include an early and marked decrease in the fasting urinary excretion of calcium. This is due to a decrease in the net release of calcium from bone and to an increase in creatinine production. The increase in creatinine output accounts for only one-third of the change, suggesting that anabolic steroids stimulate bone formation, decrease bone resorption or both.

Variable effect on bone markers

The indirect indices of skeletal turnover measured (osteocalcin, total alkaline phosphatase and hydroxyproline excretion) do not change markedly and, therefore, do not help to determine the mechanism of this effect. In one study with marked change in total activity of alkaline phosphatase, there was an increase in the bone-derived fraction.

The marked fall in fasting calcium excretion is not associated with comparable changes in serum calcium and suggests that renal tubular reabsorption of calcium is increased. No increases in serum PTH or calcitriol have, however, been reported, though urinary cAMP is increased. This suggests that anabolic steroids alter the renal sensitivity to PTH. It is thus possible that some of the skeletal effects of anabolic steroids might be mediated by an altered renal sensitivity to PTH.

EFFECTS ON BONE METABOLISM

Little is known of the mechanism of action of anabolic steroids on bone, but they may act via androgen receptors. They appear to stimulate proliferation of osteoblast-like cells *in vitro*. An increase in the bone formation rate of cancellous bone is observed and associated with an increase (albeit not significant) in the surfaces covered by active looking osteoblasts during treatment with stanozolol (Table 8.3) and suggests that the agent increases bone formation, perhaps by increasing the functional competence of osteoblasts.

Increased bone formation

The increase in the bone formation rate is associated with a comparable increase in the eroded surface and the number of osteoclasts. This suggests that stanozolol increases all the elements of bone

Table 8.3 Effects of stanozolol (mean ± SEM) on cancellous bone in patients assessed before and during continuous treatment. (From Benéton *et al.*, 1991)

	Before treatment	During treatment	Change (% pretreatment)
Bone volume (% tissue volume)	14.1 ± 1.7	14.0 ± 1.4	−1
Osteoblast surface (% bone surface)	1.08 ± 0.32	1.42 ± 0.35	+31
Osteoclast surface (% bone surface)	0.36 ± 0.13	0.49 ± 0.15	+36
Mineral apposition rate (μm/day)	0.70 ± 0.04	0.73 ± 0.05	+4
Mineralizing surface (% bone surface)	7.35 ± 1.28	14.66 ± 2.52	+99*
Bone formation rate (μm^3/μm^2/year)	19 ± 3	39 ± 7	+105†

* $P < 0.05$.
† $P < 0.02$.

Fig. 8.4 Wall thickness (mean ± SEM) in 10 patients before and during treatment with stanozolol at the sites shown. Bone structural units (BSUs) identified as formed during treatment were those bearing tetracycline labels laid down before the start of treatment. Note the significant increase in wall thickness at endocortical sites. * $P < 0.05$. (From Benéton *et al.*, 1991.)

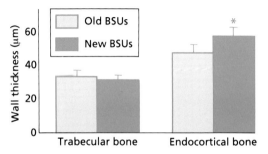

remodelling in cancellous bone. In contrast, different effects are observed at endocortical sites. The increase in the bone formation rate is not associated with any evidence of an increase in the surface of bone undergoing resorption suggesting that stanozolol increases the net apposition of bone at endocortical sites. This conclusion is supported by increases observed in wall thickness of bone structural units identified by prior tetracycline labelling as having been completed during the early phase of treatment (Fig. 8.4). The increment in wall thickness is marked (18%) and comparable to that observed in cancellous bone in patients treated with sodium fluoride. Similar findings have been observed following treatment with nandrolone (Birkenhager et al., 1990).

Effect at endocortical surface

EFFECTS ON BONE MASS

The effects of anabolic steroids on bone mass are generally consistent with a preferential effect of these agents on cortical bone sites. Treatment with methandrostenolone or with stanozolol increases total body calcium as measured by neutron-activation analysis. The increment in bone mass over the first year of treatment is similar to that over the second year which is unlike the effects of inhibitors of bone resorption (e.g., calcitonins, bisphosphonates, calcium, etc.) but more in keeping with the effects of anabolic regimens such as fluoride. Longer term studies would be required, however, to document whether steady-state conditions had been achieved.

Effects of anabolic steroids on regional skeletal sites vary according to the site and technique used. At the metacarpal, nandrolone prevents cortical bone loss (Geusens et al., 1986) consistent with a protective effect on endocortical loss. Many studies of nandrolone have shown increases in bone mass over periods of 1−2 years by absorptiometric techniques at different sites including a component of cancellous bone. These need to be interpreted cautiously because of the effects of anabolic steroids on other components of body composition (Hassager et al., 1989). They decrease the ratio of fat to lean body mass and this introduces errors into the methodology. Thus the apparent increments in BMD are due in part to these effects. Some studies suggest that the skeletal effect is the major component whereas others suggest the converse. A sustained effect on forearm bone mass has been observed by Geusens et al. (1986) for 2 years after stopping treatment with nandrolone (Fig. 8.5), whereas the effects on fat metabolism are reversed within a few months. Thus, sustained effects after stopping treatment have been attributed to treatment-induced changes in skeletal mass.

EFFECTS ON FRACTURE

There have been no prospective randomized studies to determine whether anabolic steroids reduce fracture frequency. Two studies examining the effects of stanozolol or nandrolone on bone mass

Reduced fracture frequency

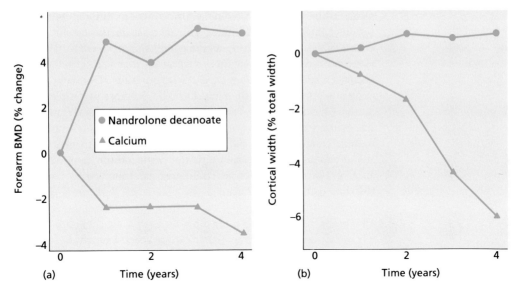

Fig. 8.5 Sequential changes in (a) forearm bone mineral density (BMD) and (b) cortical width in 9 patients given nandrolone decanoate (50 μg every 3 weeks) and in 9 patients given a calcium infusion (12 days/year; 15 mg/kg body weight per infusion). Treatment was given for 2 years. Note the apparent persistence of effect. (From Geusens *et al.*, 1986).

report fewer vertebral fractures compared with the control wing of the study. A retrospective multinational case-control study has shown that the use of anabolic steroids in women was associated with a marked (relative risk = 0.6) but not significant decrease in the relative risk of hip fracture. Analysis of these data for Italy (the country of major use) showed, however, a significant effect (Kanis *et al.*, 1993).

OTHER EFFECTS

A conspicuous effect of the anabolic steroids is to decrease fat mass and increase lean body mass, particularly muscle mass (Hassager *et al.*, 1989). This suggests that part of the beneficial effects of anabolic steroids is due to improved muscular function. Many patients report an improved mobility and greater self-confidence, and in a significant number of patients is the major benefit perceived. Other effects in osteoporotic women are an increase in skinfold thickness, perhaps due to the increased synthesis of type III collagen, a reduction in plasma fibrinogen and an increase in protein C and anti-thrombin III.

SIDE EFFECTS

Side effects, particularly hepatoxic effects are well-recognized complications of high doses of anabolic steroids as used by weightlifters and other athletes. These include peliosis hepatis (blood filled cystic lesions), hepatoma and cholestasis. These effects are not reported with the use of nandrolone or stanozolol in osteoporosis. The major side effects of their use in clinical doses vary according to the type of agent (Table 8.4).

Liver enzymes

Agents given by mouth, such as stanozolol, increase hepatic transaminases in approximately 50% of patients. These changes are reversible when treatment is stopped. Treatment is commonly continued unless liver enzyme activity exceeds two times the upper limit of the reference range. Another effect of stanozolol is the induction of an atherogenic lipid profile. This potential effect on cardiovascular risk has to be weighed against the potentially beneficial effects on coagulation, fibrinolysis and the skeleton. For this reason stanozolol and oxandrolone may be more suitable for the more elderly. A major advantage of stanozolol is that it can be given by mouth.

Virilization

Hoarseness and virilization are rare with the use of stanozolol, but is the major side effect of nandrolone which has an anabolic index 10 times lower than stanozolol. The most common side effect is hoarseness and its frequency appears to be dose-dependent. In women given 50 mg every 2 weeks, 46% of patients developed hoarseness, but is less frequent when the same dose was given at longer intervals (Need et al., 1990). For this reason, many now utilize a 4-weekly regimen and limit treatment to a year or less, but voice changes are commonly reported. Treatment-induced changes in phonation may be irreversible, but in approximately three-quarters of patients it improves following withdrawal of treatment. Changes in lipid profile are less marked than with stanozolol.

Both agents may induce mild increases in sodium retention. This is rarely a reason for stopping treatment, but diuretics may be required. Many patients report an improvement in general well being. In a few, an increase in libido is reported as an unwanted effect. Require-

Table 8.4 Advantages and disadvantages of two different anabolic steroids

	Nandrolone	Stanozolol
Hoarseness of voice	+++	+
Hirsutism	++	+
Acne	+	+
Increase in libido	+	+
Atherogenic lipid profile	+	+++
Increased hepatic transaminases	+	+++
Fluid retention	+	+
Parenteral	Yes	No

+ Occasional; ++ Uncommonly observed; +++ Commonly observed.

ments for anticoagulants and oral hypoglycaemic agents may decrease because of the effects on coagulation and glucose tolerance.

CLINICAL USE

Side effects limit use

The side effects of the anabolic steroids have limited their widespread clinical use and application. Notwithstanding, many believe that there is a place for these agents in the management of patients with

Patients feel better

osteoporosis. They are particularly suitable in the frail and elderly in whom the effects on muscle mass and self-confidence are often marked. Many patients also report improvements in back pain, even where this has been chronic. It seems likely that this is related to a change in their perception of pain, but is nevertheless a worthwhile response and has been shown objectively in a small double-blind study.

The choice of agent is more problematic. The oral agents such as stanozolol are usually given 5 mg daily on a continuous basis. In a

Choice of agent

minority of patients treatment needs to be stopped because of a reversible increase in hepatic transaminases over twice the upper limit of normal. Exceptionally, patients may need to stop treatment because of increased fluid retention or hoarseness of the voice. The optimum duration of treatment with stanozolol is not known, but the effects on cortical bone and muscle suggest that long-term treatment may be worthwhile.

The major advantage of nandrolone is its lower propensity for inducing an atherogenic lipid profile. This has to be balanced, however, against its disadvantages, which include a high frequency of hoarseness, hirsutism and other effects on virilization. A 4- or 6-weekly regimen decreases the frequency of side effects, but treatment cannot be continued indefinitely and most prefer to limit treatment to 6–12 months.

ANDROGEN THERAPY IN MEN

Androgen therapy is indicated in hypogonadal men. Testosterone by mouth or by the parenteral route is rapidly metabolized so that sustained increases in plasma levels are difficult to achieve. For this

Testosterone

reason, testosterone is commonly esterified. Testosterone propionate can be given by daily injection, but most prefer the cypionate or enanthate which are more fat soluble and undergo slower hydrolysis. Treatment with 200–300 mg by intramuscular injection is given every 2–3 weeks. The response can be monitored by the assay of testosterone and injections can be given more or less frequently to sustain testosterone levels within the normal range. Testosterone undecanoate is absorbed from the gastrointestinal tract and an adequate replacement dosage is 60 mg given twice daily. The 17-α-alkylated androgens such as methyltestosterone and methandrostenolone are also absorbed, but treatment cannot be monitored by testosterone assay. Others prefer to give testosterone implants or skin patches. The minimal effective bone-sparing dose of any of these agents is unknown.

Monitoring treatment

In primary hypogonadism it may take several weeks for plasma luteinizing hormone to decrease to the normal range. Rapid effects are observed on libido, but spermatogenesis is not restored in patients with primary hypogonadism. In primary hypogonadism it is preferable to begin treatment with small doses. Since androgens cause premature epiphyseal closure and in children may induce gynaecomastia or virilization, even when given in small amounts, treatment should not be instituted before the normal pubertal age. Feminizing side effects occur because of the conversion of testosterone to oestrogens and are more prominent in patients with hepatic cirrhosis. Other side effects include sodium retention and changes in lipid profile. The most serious complications of oral androgens are the development of peliosis hepatis and hepatoma, but these occur rarely in patients given replacement treatment. Care should be taken in patients with prostatic hypertrophy and they should be avoided in patients with prostatic cancer. Available histological evidence suggests that bone turnover (activation frequency) is decreased. However, other studies suggest that bone formation rates are increased markedly.

Delayed puberty

Delayed puberty is commonly untreated since it is considered to be a normal variant. There is, however, good evidence that it constitutes a risk for osteoporosis. Treatment is generally with the use of gonadal steroids or with anabolic steroids. These advance the timing of the growth spurt and are not thought to affect the final height attained, whereas high doses of gonadal steroids cause more rapid epiphyseal closure and can reduce the final height.

Calcitriol, alfacalcidol and related analogues

Controversial

There is probably no more controversial area in the therapeutics of osteoporosis than that concerning the use of vitamin D derivatives. The agents most widely used are calcitriol and alfacalcidol. Alfacalcidol is a synthetic analogue of calcitriol and it is metabolized to calcitriol by 25-hydroxylation in the liver. Dihydrotachysterol (DHT) has a similar structural configuration with a pseudo-1α-hydroxyl in the 3β position of the A ring. Like alfacalcidol it is metabolized in the liver to the active form 25-hydroxy-dihydrotachysterol. Experience with its use alone in uncomplicated osteoporosis is limited and DHT has been largely used in combination with fluoride. The use of parent vitamin D in osteoporosis is discussed in Chapter 9.

Both alfacalcidol and calcitriol are licensed for use in several countries, but licences have also been refused in others. The greatest use occurs in Japan and many studies, particularly those with alfacalcidol, have been undertaken in Japan.

METABOLIC EFFECTS

Doses of calcitriol used in osteoporosis have ranged from 250 ng to 1 µg daily given either as a single daily dose or twice daily. Somewhat larger doses have been used for alfacalcidol since the potency of alfacalcidol is approximately half that of calcitriol. Both are given as continuous regimens. Their administration leads to a sustained dose-dependent increase in the intestinal absorption of calcium. As might be expected, increased circulating concentrations of calcitriol with the use of calcitriol or alfacalcidol are associated with increased concentrations of osteocalcin, an increase in serum calcium and a decrease in PTH. Longer term effects are consistent with a primary effect to decrease bone resorption. Most studies show a dose-dependent decrease in the urinary excretion of hydroxyproline. Similarly, low doses of alfacalcidol or calcitriol have little effect on total activity of alkaline phosphatase but activity decreases with higher doses. As expected, the urinary excretion of calcium is increased.

Dose-dependent effects

The most conspicuous effect, therefore, of both calcitriol and alfacalcidol is to increase the intestinal absorption of calcium, raise serum calcium and reduce the secretion of PTH. In this way it is likely to decrease bone remodelling in much the same way as is observed with pharmacological doses of calcium. The major difference between the use of vitamin D derivatives and the use of calcium is that in the former, serum calcitriol levels will be high whereas in the latter they will be low. The question arises, therefore, whether there are particular effects of vitamin D on bone formation or quality, a subject that has intrigued investigators for more than 40 years.

Does it differ from calcium?

EFFECTS ON BONE MASS

Many studies have been reported on the effects of both alfacalcidol and calcitriol on bone mass. Some have been comparative studies with other treatments or not randomly assigned to treatment and control wings. Others have been more adequately controlled and are discussed below.

Variable response

The response observed to treatment has been remarkably heterogeneous (Table 8.5). Some investigators have shown very large increments in skeletal mass over short periods of time in the order of 10–20%. This is likely to reflect the healing of coexisting osteomalacia. Other investigators have shown more modest increases in bone mineral which subsequently declined in magnitude (Fig. 8.6) as might be expected of a primary effect to inhibit bone resorption. Others, however, have shown no effect. An increase in cortical width has not been observed.

Several explanations have been offered for the variable responses observed. The first is that the requirements for calcitriol vary according to the nutritional status for calcium. The argument runs that women with a low calcium intake are calcium deficient and it is these patients that would respond. Although the rationale behind this

Table 8.5 Reported effects of calcitriol on bone mass in postmenopausal osteporosis

Study design*	Average dose (ng/day)	Patients (number)	Treatment duration (months)	Technique applied†	Site‡	Effect§	Source
D	800	27	24	NAA	TB	++	Aloia et al. (1988)
				SPA	FA	++	
D	620	40	24	DPA	LS	++	Gallagher & Riggs (1990)
				DPA	TB	++	
				DPA	Head	++	
				MCI	Hand	−	
D	1000‖	37	4	SPA	FA	0	Hoikka et al. (1980)
D	250‖	264	24	SPA	FA	0	Christiansen et al. (1980)
D	250	48	12	SPA	FA	−	Christiansen et al. (1981)
D	500	74	12	SPA	UDR	0	Jensen et al. (1982)
				SPA	FA	−	
S	500	76	36	DPA	FA	+	Falch et al. (1987)
D	1000‖	300	6	XRD	Hand	++	Fujita et al. (1990)

* D, double blind; S, single blind.
† NAA, neutron activation analysis; MCI, metacarpal index; SPA, single photon absorptiometry; DPA, dual photon absorptiometry; XRD, X-ray density.
‡ TB, total body; FA, forearm; LS, lumbar spine; UDR, ultradistal radius.
§ In comparison with controls: −accelerated loss; 0, no difference; +, small difference; ++, significant difference.
‖ Alfacalcidol.

argument can be questioned, it is nevertheless possible that, if calcitriol has direct effects on bone rather than only through an effect on serum calcium, those on a high calcium diet become hypercalcaemic more readily, and therefore tolerate lower doses of calcitriol. A further explanation, perhaps more plausible, is that the therapeutic window

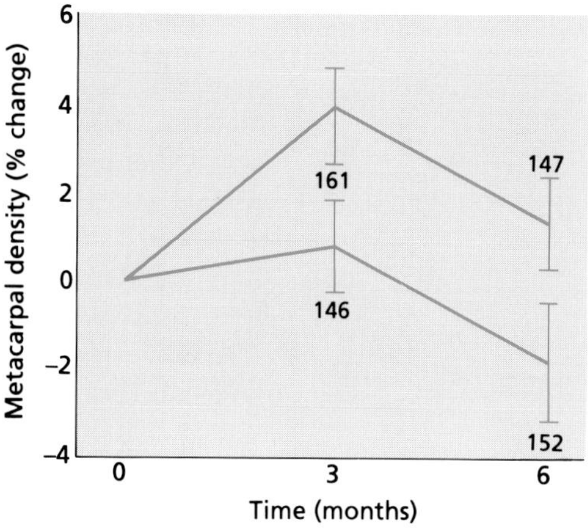

Fig. 8.6 Short-term effects of alfacalcidol or placebo on mineral density (mean ± SEM) at the metacarpal in patients with osteoporosis. Numbers refer to the sample size at each time. (From Fujita et al., 1990.)

for calcitriol is narrow and the response in a population to a fixed dose is heterogeneous. Thus, a dose which is beneficial for some is toxic for others. Finally, it is argued that, because some patients have end-organ resistance to vitamin D, positive responses can only be expected in those patients where such defects contribute to the pathophysiology of their osteoporosis. A further factor likely to account for variable responses is variable degrees of occult vitamin D deficiency.

EFFECTS ON FRACTURE

There have been several prospective and randomized studies which have examined the effects of calcitriol on vertebral fracture rates (Table 8.6). The effects reported are as heterogeneous as those reported on bone mass. Some show a significant effect and others no effect on vertebral fracture risk.

The majority of the studies reported have characterized a new vertebral fracture as a 15% or greater decrease in vertebral height. This is likely to have introduced a large number of false-positives to the apparent rate of fractures, which would decrease the magnitude of any apparent effect and might also influence the direction of effects (see Chapter 7). It is possible, therefore, that beneficial effects of calcitriol occurred but were missed. Thus, the negative studies as presented are not helpful and the studies showing beneficial effects should be examined.

In this regard, the two trials showing the greatest effect of calcitriol have been those of Tilyard (Tilyard *et al.*, 1992) on large numbers of

Table 8.6 Randomized prospective studies of the effects of calcitriol on vertebral fracture

Study duration (months)	Dose of calcitriol (ng/day)	Study design*	Patients enrolled†	Percent completing	Calcium intake test wing (mg/day)	Relative risk of fracture	Source
12	500	D	62	87	700	0.47	Gallagher & Riggs (1990)
12	400	D	58	71	500	1.0‡	Jensen et al. (1985)
24	800	D	37	79	250–500	0.75	Aloia et al. (1988)
24	430	D	86	84	600	2.22	Ott & Chestnut (1989)
24	620	D	50	80	600	1.16	Gallagher & Riggs (1990)
36	500	O	515	83	885	0.31§	Tilyard et al. (1992)

* D, double blind; O, open randomized.
† Test and control wings.
‡ No effect on spine score.
§ Significantly decreased.

patients and that of Gallagher & Riggs (1990) on a more modest number (see Table 8.6). In the latter study, patients were enrolled into a 3-year study but were allocated to calcitriol or placebo only for 1 year. During this year of intervention, vertebral fracture frequency decreased from 823/1000 patient years in the placebo treated wing to 450/1000 patient years in the test wing.

Variable results

These findings contrast markedly with the results of the study published by Tilyard *et al.* (1992) which was a prospective randomized but open study undertaken in New Zealand in more than 600 post-menopausal women. The vertebral fracture rate did not decrease in the first year of treatment. Thereafter, there was a significant difference in fracture rate between patients given calcitriol and those given calcium (Table 8.7). There is, however, a problem in the interpretation of this study in that it is to be expected that vertebral fracture frequency will decrease with time. The fracture rate remained constant, however, in patients allocated to calcitriol. The difference in trial outcome, therefore, resulted from an increase in vertebral fracture frequency with the use of calcium. The rather devastating conclusion that might be drawn from this study is that calcitriol prevented calcium-induced vertebral fractures! The explanation for the effect is not obvious, but the interpretation that calcitriol decreases the risk of fracture on the basis of the reported results is questionable.

More consistent effects of alfacalcidol

The effects of alfacalcidol on vertebral fracture frequency appear to be much more consistent but are all based on open studies. Several open but randomized trials have demonstrated a significant effect of alfacalcidol alone or in combination with eel calcitonin or calcium

Table 8.7 Effects of calcitriol (250 ng twice daily) or calcium (1 g daily) on vertebral fracture frequency. (From Tilyard *et al.*, 1992)

	Calcitriol	Calcium
From enrolment to 1 year		
Number of patients	262	253
Patients with new fractures	14	17
Number of new fractures	23	26
Fracture rate/100 patient years	88	103
Year 1 to year 2		
Number of patients	232	240
Patients with new fractures	14	30
Number of new fractures	24	60
Fracture rate/100 patient years	99	250
Year 2 to 3		
Number of patients	213	219
Patients with new fractures	12	44
Number of new fractures	21	69
Fracture rate/100 patient years	99	315

on fracture rates (Fig. 8.7). The largest study undertaken with alfa-calcidol was on 666 patients enrolled into an open but randomized study for 1 year (Hayashi *et al.*, 1992). A dose of 1 µg was given daily without calcium supplements and was associated with a significantly lower vertebral fracture frequency compared to those not given treatment (76 vs 41/100 patient years). It is of interest that these positive outcomes in the case of alfacalcidol were all undertaken in Japan where the customary intake of calcium is low. This accords with an extraordinarily low incidence of hypercalcaemia reported in Japan.

No studies have been undertaken to examine the effects of alfa-calcidol or calcitriol on hip fracture. A retrospective case-control study showed no significant effect of vitamin D products on the risk of hip fracture, but the type of agent used was not known (Kanis *et al.*, 1992).

SIDE EFFECTS
With the average Western diet, hypercalcaemia is common. The adverse effects of prolonged hypercalcaemia are well recognized and include impairment of renal function and nephrocalcinosis. One study has reported impaired renal function, but this has not been confirmed. When hypercalcaemia was avoided one study reported a small and reversible decrease in glomerular filtration rate not shown by others. On the other hand, serum creatinine may rise for other reasons. No long-term adverse effects are reported in the absence of hyper-calcaemia. In contrast to vitamin D toxicity with the parent compound, the rate of onset and reversal of hypercalcaemia with the 1α-hydroxylated derivatives is significantly more rapid (Kanis & Russell, 1977). The major advantage of this rapid effect is that it permits the flexible titration of dose to requirements. The narrow therapeutic window nevertheless demands that frequent surveillance of serum and possibly urinary calcium should be undertaken in patients exposed to these agents.

Hypercalcaemia

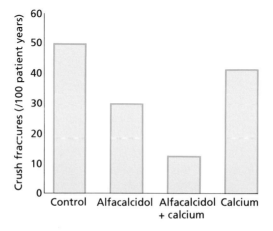

Fig. 8.7 Effects of alfacalcidol, calcium and the combination on vertebral fracture frequency. (From Orimo et al. 1987.)

OTHER VITAMIN D DERIVATIVES

A number of other derivatives of vitamin D have been tested in osteoporosis. These include 1α-hydroxyvitamin D_2, 1,24-dihydroxy-vitamin D and 24,25-dihydroxyvitamin D (secalciferol). 1,24(OH)$_2$D$_3$ is less potent than calcitriol, but there is little evidence to date that apart from the dose needed, there is any difference in the therapeutic window or spectrum of response. Secalciferol has also been tested in osteoporosis. Physiologically appropriate doses acutely increase calcium retention in patients with osteoporosis, but this is ill sustained. Very high pharmacological doses, however, increase bone mass markedly in experimental animals and the use of higher doses is presently being studied in humans.

Thiazide diuretics

The actions of thiazide diuretics are complex but the major effect on skeletal metabolism in humans is probably mediated by their ability to increase renal tubular reabsorption of calcium under steady-state conditions. The ultimate effect is to increase serum calcium, lower PTH and calcitriol, and decrease both the intestinal absorption of calcium and bone turnover. There may however be additional direct effects of thiazides on bone and intestine.

Many studies suggest that the use of thiazides should be considered in the management of osteoporosis. Population studies have indicated that patients receiving thiazides have a higher bone mineral than those who do not. A longitudinal observational study reported that men taking thiazides for hypertension had a significantly slower rate of loss than those taking other antihypertensive drugs (Wasnich *et al.*, 1990). A variety of case-control studies have shown the use of thiazides to be associated with a significantly decreased risk of hip fracture. Similar results were shown in a cohort study. However, a recent case-control study showed a significant increase in risk. Despite the wealth of epidemiological data there are few prospective randomized studies and none which examine fracture rates.

Slows rate of bone loss

Exercise

Exercise regimens can be very helpful in the management of established osteoporosis. Whereas there are perhaps minor gains to be achieved in terms of skeletal mass (see Chapter 6), there are major benefits for self-confidence and a sense of well-being. In addition, physiotherapy and simple postural advice can commonly help chronic pain. Management of patients with kyphosis includes attention to posture while standing, sitting and lying. Sitting with a cushion behind the neck may be helpful in the presence of kyphosis. Most patients with vertebral osteoporosis get relief from bed rest particularly with a firm rather than soft mattress. Neck pillows are also helpful.

Good for well-being

Many people are reluctant to advise more active exercise for osteoporotic patients because of concerns about further fractures. Clearly immobility will worsen the situation and violent activity will increase the risks. There is a good case, however, for taking the middle ground. Exercises carefully structured according to the disability of the patient improve not only well-being and confidence, but also improve postural stability. Some centres have set up dedicated exercise programmes for patients with vertebral osteoporosis with supervised exercise classes twice weekly (Harrison *et al.*, 1993). Their initial and subsequent performance was evaluated annually. The compliance was 56% over a 4-year interval. Although this was not a randomized study, an analysis of those who attained greatest fitness during the programme showed a significant decrease in back pain score and a trend to fewer further fractures (Table 8.8).

In patients with vertebral osteoporosis, loads on the anterior aspect of the vertebral bodies should be avoided. Indeed, exercise programmes which include flexion activity increase the risk of new vertebral fractures compared to a programme of progressive resistance exercises, which strengthen the extensor muscles of the back (Sinaki & Mikkelsen, 1984). Walking, cycling, dancing (according to preference) and swimming (particularly in adequately heated water) provide excellent exercise for most patients. These can be incorporated with hydrotherapy exercise. Patients should be discouraged from exercise programmes not initiated under the supervision of a trained physiotherapist and tailored to the patient. Commercial video tapes, unless dedicated to patients with osteoporosis, should be avoided.

Treatment of falls

With the exception of vertebral fractures, the vast majority of fragility fractures occur after falls. The risk of falling increases with age and is greater in women than in men. Approximately one-third of elderly individuals over the age of 65 years fall each year. This suggests that treatment of falls, if feasible, might have a marked impact on the frequency of fracture. A variety of studies have indicated the risk

Table 8.8 Effect of an exercise programme in osteoporotic patients according to the degree of fitness achieved (as assessed by maximal oxygen uptake). (From Harrison *et al.*, 1993)

	Less fit	More fit	P
Number of patients	36	37	
Improvement in back pain score (% initial value ± SEM)	11.7 ± 16	32.8 ± 11	0.03
Number of new vertebral fractures	10	3	0.09
Number of new non-vertebral fractures	16	13	NS

factors associated with falls (Table 8A). With the possible exception of the use of long-acting barbiturates the major factors relate to coexistent morbidity which is mainly irreversible. Well-intentioned

Difficult to prevent falls

environmental advice may in fact be counterproductive since a change in environment may also cause falls. There is thus little evidence that falls can indeed be prevented (Perry, 1992; Vetter *et al.*, 1992). Notwithstanding, in individual patients, causes can sometimes be identified. In one randomized controlled prospective study, elderly patients in residential care were examined and counselled following a fall in the one wing, whereas in the other wing no intervention was undertaken. Attention was paid to risk factors such as postural hypotension and side effects of drugs. After 2 years the intervention wing had significantly fewer hospitalizations. Although there was a 9% decrease in the frequency of falls this was not significant.

Given the fall there are a number of factors which might increase the risk of fracture resulting from a fall. Falling directly on the hip

Use of hip protectors

increases the risk markedly. Falling onto a hard surface and the presence of reduced soft tissue padding also increase the risk. Recently, a randomized study was undertaken in a nursing home environment where patients were allocated to wear a padded propylene external hip protector, whereas the other wing were untreated. Hip fractures were significantly less frequent in the treatment wing (Table 8.9). This suggests that the use of external protectors may be of value, particularly in the nursing home environment where the age-specific risk is substantially greater than that in the general community.

Table 8A Causes of falling in the elderly

> *Drugs*
> Hypnotics, minor and major tranquillizers
> Alcohol
> Loop diuretics and hypotensive agents, inducing postural hypotension
> Hypoglycaemic agents
> Digoxin and dysrhythmia inducing agents
>
> *Diseases*
> Cerebrovascular: stroke, transient ischaemic attacks, postural
>   hypotension, vertebrobasilar insufficiency, dysrhythmias
> Neurological: senile dementia, Parkinson's disease, autonomic
>   neuropathy, abnormal frontal lobe reflexes
> Impaired vision, e.g., cataract
>
> *Environmental*
> Slippery surfaces
> Loose wires and rugs
> Snow and ice
> Inadequate walking aids
> Unfamiliar environment

Table 8.9 Effect of wearing an external hip protector in nursing home residents on the risk of hip fracture. (From Lauritzen et al., 1993)

	Hip protector	No protector	Relative risk (95% confidence intervals)
Number of patients	247	418	
Number of hip fractures (%)	8 (3.2)*	31 (7.4)	0.44 (0.21−0.94)
Number of non-hip fractures (%)	15 (6.1)	27 (6.5)	0.94 (0.51−1.7)
Hip fractures/fall on hip %†	8.3	26.3	

* None of the patients were wearing a protector at the time of the fall.
† Estimated in a sample of patients.

Experimental drug regimens

A great variety of combinations, sequential and intermittent regimens have been studied. Some have been previously mentioned such as the sequential use of phosphate and etidronate. Others include PTH combined with calcitonin, growth hormone with calcitonin, calcitriol and clodronate, and oestrogens with anabolic steroids or fluoride to name but a few. Whether any will be of ultimate benefit is not known. There are several experimental agents which may be of interest in the future (Table 8.10). Of these, the greatest amount of work has been done on ipriflavone, a synthetic flavinoid. Indeed the agent is available in Italy, Belgium and Japan for the management of osteoporosis. It appears to inhibit bone resorption in oophorectomized

Table 8.10 Experimental drug regimens for osteoporosis tested in humans

Combination and sequential regimens	Single agents
Calcitonin with phosphate	PTH
PTH	Vitamin K_2
Thyroxine	Tamoxifen and related agents
Growth hormone	Growth hormone
PTH with oestrogens	Strontium
Anabolic steroids	Aluminium salts
Calcitriol	Silicates
Growth hormone	Ipriflavone
Growth hormone with calcitonin	Raloxifene
Clodronate with calcitriol	
Oestrogens with anabolic steroids	Promethazine
H$_2$-receptor antagonists	
Fluoride with oestrogens	

PTH, parathyroid hormone.

women and in postmenopausal osteoporosis and may also potentiate the effect of exogenous or endogenous oestrogens on bone. Raloxifene is currently undergoing extensive clinical testing both for prevention and treatment. Other single agents include the bisphosphonates alendronate, tiludronate and clodronate, and the antihistamine promethazine.

Management of established osteoporosis

The management of osteoporosis includes not only the maintenance of skeletal mass, but also the management of symptomatic disease and its consequences. The orthopaedic management of fractures is beyond the scope of this volume but there are a number of considerations which relate to the medical rather than surgical care of established osteoporosis. With the exception of vertebral fractures, surgical management is generally preferable in the elderly, where feasible, because of the increased morbidity including bone loss that is associated with immobilization.

Diet

Many hospital diets are inadequate in terms of nutritional requirements for the elderly, and in a controlled prospective study, both complications and deaths were significantly decreased in patients with hip fracture who were provided a nutritional supplement (Delmi et al., 1990).

The frequency and severity of symptoms in acute vertebral fracture vary enormously and so, therefore, do the aims of acute management. At best, they are asymptomatic and at worst give rise to acute disabling pain at the site with intense pain which may be exacerbated by trivial movements such as deep breathing or coughing (see Chapter 1). Thus, one of the major aims of acute treatment is to relieve pain and restore daily activities as soon as possible. Spinal compression fractures are most painful in flexion and aggravated by standing. Acute pain may require opiates for a day or so, though where possible these should be avoided. Mobilization should be feasible within a week or two at the most. The mobilization programme should be as rapid as possible, consistent with the general clinical state of the patient and the degree of residual pain. Continuous bed rest should obviously be for as brief a period as possible and, if inevitable, the use of an inhibitor of bone resorption should be considered. Calcitonin in this regard is attractive because of its added effects on analgesia. Etidronate should probably not be given but other bisphosphonates are not contraindicated. Their effects on acute pain have not yet been adequately tested.

Acute management

Regain maximal function

A period of limited mobilization thereafter should gradually evolve towards attaining maximal function over the next few months during which the patient should be encouraged to return to many of the usual activities at home, using a lumbar support or extension brace where appropriate, and brief periods of intermittent bed rest. Mild sedation may diminish the paravertebral muscle spasm and pain may additionally be relieved by heat or by ice. Most patients are free of local pain after 2–3 months, but during this time there is risk of developing postural low back pain due to the redistribution of weight.

Pain

Continued pain may be relieved by non-steroidal anti-inflammatory agents and the use of a spinal support. In general the higher the vertebral level which is fractured the less satisfactory the results. It is, however, difficult to predict who will benefit from spinal supports. Probably the best way to utilize these are to offer them where necessary but to tell the patient to discard this if no relief is obtained. During this subacute phase, intermittent periods of bed rest throughout the day may be helpful. The use of foam inserts to cushion the effects of walking may also improve mobility. In the elderly a walking stick or Zimmer frame may provide extra support to help patients mobilize with confidence.

After the acute phase, isometric exercises may be very helpful. Again, it is difficult to predict who will or who will not improve from treatment. As mentioned, it is important that exercise programmes are geared towards the patient and are not too ambitious. Twisting of the torso or lifting with flexion should be avoided. Some patients, particularly those with muscle pain, get relief from heat pads or from heat or infrared lamps. Others find ice pads helpful. Transcutaneous electric nerve stimulators can also be helpful. Other techniques such as acupuncture or yoga should only be contemplated with experienced practitioners who have a knowledge of osteoporosis.

Persistent symptoms

Some patients have persistent back pain most often related to the deformities and the stress this puts on the adjacent muscles and joints. The same aspects of management, namely pain relief, attention to posture, spinal supports and physical exercises, are important. Instruction on lifting techniques and bending should be given in order to avoid undue stresses. There is an important role for exercise in the management of chronic vertebral osteoporosis and in the chronic management of hip fracture. This relates more to the effects of exercise on physical fitness, balance and confidence than on any effects on bone mass.

Treatment and fracture healing

Questions arise whether medical treatment affects the healing fracture. Apparently normal rates of fracture healing have been observed in patients given either calcitonin or clodronate immediately before fracture or throughout conservative management of long-bone fractures. In experimental animals calcitonin may indeed accelerate fracture repair. In the case of the bisphosphonates no impairment of fracture healing or the strength of callus has been observed, but the resorption of callus is delayed. An exception is that large doses of etidronate impair fracture healing in humans as do lower doses in experimental animals. This suggests that etidronate should be stopped if long-bone fractures occur. The occurrence of long-bone fractures in patients treated with sodium fluoride should

Table 8.11 Comparative properties of commonly used drug treatments for established osteoporosis

Feature	Agent							
	Calcium ± vitamin D	Vitamin D analogues	Gonadal steroids	Calcitonins	Etidronate	Other bisphosphonates	Anabolic steroids	Fluorides
Long-term compliance	High	Unknown	Poor	Variable*	Unknown	Unknown	High	Moderate
Side effects	Rare	Variable	Common	Variable*	Occasional	Occasional	Common	Common
Effects on cancellous bone mass	Modest	Modest	Marked	Proven	Proven†	Proven	Moderate	Substantial
Effect on cortical thickness	Modest	None	Established	Variable‡	Not known	Unknown	Established	Modest
Effect on vertebral fracture	Modest	Variable	Proven	Probable	Possible	Probable	Probable	Moderate
Effects on hip fracture	Probable	Unproven	Proven	Probable	Unknown	Unknown	Probable	None
Extraskeletal benefits	None	None	Cardiovascular	Analgesic	None	None	Muscle mass	None
Duration of treatment (years)	Indefinite	Uncertain	10	5	Up to 3	Uncertain	1–5*	1–5
Offset of effect on stopping treatment	Rapid	Rapid	Rapid	Rapid	Slow	Slow	?Rapid	?Slow

* Depends on formulation.
† Long-term effects (>5 years not known).
‡ Dose uncertain.

also be a reason for stopping treatment since fluoride will be taken up avidly at the site of fracture.

With the bewildering array of medical interventions, the question arises which agent should be used under which circumstances in patients with established osteoporosis. Some of the comparative aspects of the agents commonly utilized are summarized in Table 8.11. They all have advantages and disadvantages. In younger women who have had fractures hormone replacement therapy should certainly be discussed. As reviewed, the uptake and long-term compliance with hormone replacement therapy is limited and there is, therefore, a place for other interventions, even if their efficacy is less complete or less secure. Neither etidronate nor fluoride should be given to patients with hip fracture, and we avoid the use of fluoride in patients with markedly reduced decreases in cortical width. In several countries, calcitonin is only available as a parenteral formulation and this poses problems with its long-term use. Some treatments require more supervision than others and the less supervision required the more a person treated will not feel like a patient. In the vast majority of cases a consideration of the advantages and disadvantages of each treatment modality results in a clear therapeutic strategy.

References

Aaron JE, de Vernejoul MC, Kanis JA (1991) The effect of sodium fluoride on trabecular architecture in osteoporosis. *Bone*; **12**: 307–310.

Aloia JF, Waswani A, Yeh JK *et al.* (1988) Calcitriol in the treatment of post-menopausal osteoporosis. *Am J Med*; **84**: 401–408.

Baylink DJ, Bernstein DS (1967) The effect of fluoride therapy on metabolic bone disease: a histologic study. *Clin Orthop*; **55**: 51–85.

Benéton MNC, Yates AJP, Rogers S *et al.* (1991) Stanozolol stimulates remodelling of trabecular bone and the net formation of bone at the endocortical surface. *Clin Sci*; **81**: 543–549.

Birkenhager JC, v Huijk C, Erdtsieck RJ *et al.* (1990) Effect of HRT and HRT plus nandrolone in postmenopausal osteoporosis (PMO): an interim analysis. In Christiansen C, Overgaard K (eds). *Osteoporosis*, pp. 1363–1365. Osteopress, Copenhagen.

Briancon D, Meunier P (1979) Le traitement de l'osteoporose par l'association fluorure de sodium, calcium, vitamine D. Thesis, Lyon.

Briancon D, Meunier PJ (1981) Treatment of osteoporosis with fluoride, calcium and vitamin D. *Orth Clin N Am*; **12**: 629–648.

Buckle RM (1989) 3-year study of sodium fluoride treatment on vertebral fracture incidence in osteoporosis. *J Bone Miner Res*; **4** (suppl. 1): S186.

Christiansen C, Christensen MS, McNair P *et al.* (1980) Prevention of early post-menopausal bone loss controlled 2-year study in 315 normal females. *Eur J Clin Invest*; **10**. 273–279.

Christiansen C, Christensen MS, Rodbro P *et al.* (1981) Effect of 1,25-dihydroxy-vitamin D_3 in itself or combined with hormone treatment in preventing post-menopausal osteoporosis. *Eur J Clin Invest*; **11**: 305–309.

Dambacher MA, Lauffenburger T, Lammble B, Haas HG (1978) Long-term effects of sodium fluoride in osteoporosis. In Courvoisier B, Donath A (eds). *Fluoride* and Bone, pp. 238–241. Hans Huber, Bern.

Delmi M, Rapin C-H, Bengoa J-M et al. (1990) Dietary supplementation in elderly patients with fractured neck of the femur. Lancet; **335**: 1013–1016.

Ekstrand J, Ehrnebo M, Boreus LO (1978) Fluoride bioavailability after intravenous and oral administration: importance of renal clearance and urine flow. Clin Pharmacol Ther; **23**: 329–337.

Eriksen EF, Mosekilde L, Melsen F (1985) Effects of sodium fluoride, calcium phosphate and vitamin D_2 on bone balance and remodelling in osteoporotics. Bone; **6**: 381–390.

Falch JA, Odeggard OR, Finnager AM, Mathëson I (1987) Postmenopausal osteoporosis: no effect of three years treatment with 1,25-dihydroxycholecalciferol. Acta Med Scand; **221**: 199–204.

Farley JR, Wergedal JE, Baylink DJ (1983) Fluoride directly stimulates proliferation and alkaline phosphatase activity of bone forming cells. Science; **222**: 330–332.

Farley SM, Wergedal JE, Farley JR et al. (1992) Spinal fractures during fluoride therapy for osteoporosis: relationship to spinal bone density. Osteoporosis Int; **2**: 213–218.

Fujita T, Matsui T, Nakao Y et al. (1990) Cytokines and osteoporosis. Ann NY Acad Sci; **587**: 371–375.

Gallagher JC, Riggs BL (1990) Action of 1,25-dihydroxyvitamin D_3 on calcium balance and bone turnover and its effects on vertebral fracture rate. Metabolism; **4** (suppl. 1): 30–34.

Geusens P, Dequeker J, Verstraeten A et al. (1986) Bone mineral content, cortical thickness and fracture rate in osteoporotic women after withdrawal of treatment with nandrolone decanoate, 1-alpha hydroxyvitamin D_3 or intermittent calcium infusions. Maturitas; **8**: 281–289.

Harrison JE, McNeil KG, Sturtridge WC et al. (1981) Three year changes in bone mineral mass of postmenopausal osteoporotic patients based on neutron activation analysis of the central third of the skeleton. J Clin Endocr Metab; **52**: 751–758.

Harrison JE, Chow R, Dornan J et al. (1993) Evaluation of a program for rehabilitation of osteoporotic patients (PRO): 4-year follow-up. Osteoporosis Int; **3**: 13–17.

Hassager C, Podenphant J, Riis BJ et al. (1989) Changes in soft tissue body composition and plasma lipid metabolism during androlone decanoate therapy in postmenopausal osteoporotic women. Metab Clin Exp; **38**: 238–242.

Hayashi Y, Fujita T, Inoue T (1992) Decrease of vertebral fracture in osteoporotics by administration of 1α-hydroxy-vitamin D_3. J Bone Miner Metab; **10**: 50(184)–54(188).

Hoikka V, Ahlava EM, Aro A et al. (1980) Treatment of osteoporosis with 1-alpha-hydroxycholecalciferol and calcium. Acta Med Scand; **207**: 221–224.

Jensen GF, Christiansen C, Transbol I (1982) Treatment of postmenopausal osteoporosis. A controlled therapeutic trial comparing oestrogen/gestagen, 1,25-dihydroxyvitamin D_3 and calcium. Clin Endocrinol; **16**: 515–524.

Jensen GF, Meinecke B, Boesen J, Tansbol I (1985) Does 1,25(OH)$_2$D$_3$ accelerate spinal bone loss? A controlled therapeutic trial on 70-year-old women. Clin Orthop; **192**: 215–221.

Kanis JA, Russell RGG (1977) Rate of reversal of hypercalcaemia induced by vitamin D_3 and its 1α-hydroxylated derivatives. BMJ; **i**: 78–81.

Kanis JA, Meunier PJ (1984) Should we use fluoride to treat osteoporosis? Quart J Med; **53**: 145–164.

Kanis JA, Johnell O, Gullberg B et al. (1992) Evidence for the efficacy of bone active drugs in the prevention of hip fracture. BMJ; **305**: 1124–1128.

Kanis JA, Benéton MNC, Gennari C et al. (1993) Effects of anabolic steroids on cortical bone and fractures. In Christiansen C, Overgaard K (eds). Osteoporosis

1993, pp. 308–310. Osteopress, Copenhagen.

Kleerekoper M, Peterson EL, Nelson DA *et al.* (1990) A randomized trial of sodium fluoride as a treatment for postmenopausal osteoporosis. *Osteoporosis Int*; **1**: 155–161.

Lauritzen JB, Petersen MM, Lund B (1993) Effect of external hip protectors on hip fractures. *Lancet*; **341**: 11–13.

Mamelle N, Meunier PJ, Dusan R *et al.* (1988) Risk–benefit ratio of sodium fluoride: treatment in primary vertebral osteoporosis. *Lancet*; **ii**: 361–365.

Merz W (1981) The essential trace elements. *Science*; **213**: 1332–1338.

Nagant de Deuxchaisnes C, Devogelaer JP, Stein F (1990) Comparison of the bioavailability of the NaF capsules used in the NIH-sponsored trials as compared to that of NaF enteric-coated tablets commercially available in Europe. *J Bone Miner Res*; **5** (suppl. 2): S251.

Need AG, Durbridge TC, Nordin BEC (1990) Anabolic steroids. In: Kanis JA (ed.). Calcium Metabolism, pp. 165–182. Kager, Basel.

Orimo H, Shiraki M, Hayashi T *et al.* (1987) Reduced occurrence of vertebral crush fractures in senile osteoporosis treated with 1(OH)-vitamin D_3. *Bone Miner*; **3**: 47–52.

Ott S, Chestnut CH (1989) Calcitriol treatment is not effective in postmenopausal osteoporosis. *Ann Intern Med*; **110**: 267–274.

Parsons V, Mitchell C, Eimond A, Darby AJ (1983) The use of sodium fluoride and calcium supplements and vitamin D in the treatment of axial osteoporosis. In Dixon A, StJ, Russell RGG, Stamp TCB (eds). *Osteoporosis, a Multidisciplinary Problem*, pp. 259–264. Royal Society of Medicine and Academic Press, London.

Perry BC (1992) Falls among the elderly: a review of the methods and conclusions of epidemiologic studies. *J Am Geriatr Soc*; **30**: 367–371.

Riggs BL, Seeman E, Hodgson SF *et al.* (1982) Effect of the fluoride/calcium regimen on vertebral fracture occurrence in postmenopausal osteoporosis. Comparison with conventional therapy. *N Engl J Med*; **306**: 446–450.

Riggs BL, Baylink DJ, Kleerekoper M *et al.* (1987) Incidence of hip fractures in osteoporotic women treated with sodium fluoride. *J Bone Miner Res*; **2**: 123–126.

Riggs BL, Hodgson SF, O'Fallon WM *et al.* (1990) Effect of fluoride treatment on the fracture rate in postmenopausal women with osteoporosis. *N Engl J Med*; **22**: 802–809.

Riggs BL, O'Fallon WM, Lane A *et al.* (1994) Clinical trial of fluoride therapy in postmenopausal osteoporotic women: extended observations and additional analysis. *J Bone Miner Res*; **9**: 265–275.

Schnitzler CM (1984) Stress fractures in fluoride therapy for osteoporosis. In Christiansen C, Argand CD, Nordin BEC *et al.* (eds). *Osteoporosis*, pp. 629–634. Glostrup Hospital, Denmark.

Sinaki M, Mikkelsen BA (1984) Postmenopausal spinal osteoporosis: flexion versus extension exercises. *Arch Phys Med Rehab*; **65**: 593–596.

Tilyard M, Spears GFS, Thomson J, Dovey S (1992) Treatment of postmenopausal osteoporosis with calcitriol or calcium. *N Engl J Med*; **326**: 357–362.

Vetter NJ, Lewis PA, Ford D (1992) Can health visitors prevent fractures in elderly people? *BMJ*; **304**: 888–890.

Vose GP, Keele DK, Milner AM *et al.* (1978) Effect of sodium fluoride, inorganic phosphate and oxymetholone therapies in osteoporosis: a six year progress report. *J Gerontol*; **33**: 204–212.

Wasnich R, Davis J, Ross P, Vogel J (1990) Effect of thiazide on rates of bone mineral loss: a longitudinal study. *BMJ*; **301**: 1303–1305.

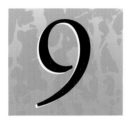

9 Treatment of secondary and focal osteoporosis

Reversal of contributory factors

It is perhaps obvious that the management of all forms of osteoporosis demands a consideration of its pathophysiology to reverse, if possible, some of the contributory factors. With regard to secondary osteoporosis, treatment of the cause may in many cases halt or, more rarely, reverse the osteoporotic process. Many of the factors causing secondary osteoporosis are reviewed in Chapter 4 and in several instances additional aspects of their management are provided or are obvious. In other instances the treatment of the disorder is similar to that outlined in Chapters 6–8. There are, however, additional aspects of the management of several secondary causes of osteoporosis which are reviewed below. In addition, the experience in treatment with bone-active drugs is much more limited than in uncomplicated osteoporosis so that a review of interventions tested in these secondary causes of osteoporosis is appropriate.

Management of secondary causes of osteoporosis

Corticosteroid-induced osteoporosis

Difficult to study

Corticosteroid-induced osteoporosis is probably the most important secondary cause of osteoporosis, but it has been a relatively neglected area of therapeutic research, partly because of the heterogeneous nature of the underlying disorders for which corticosteroids are utilized. Notwithstanding, many studies have been undertaken, usually on relatively small sample sizes, examining the effects of either stimulators of bone formation or inhibitors of bone resorption on bone mass. Few studies have assessed the effects of intervention on fracture rates.

> As in the case of all causes of osteoporosis, the aims of treatment are to reduce symptoms, where present, by adequate medication, maintain and maximize mobility and to prevent or treat osteoporosis.

Monitor bone mass

The frequency of osteoporosis and fractures is sufficiently great that patients who are committed to long-term corticosteroids should be assessed for osteoporosis and, if intervention is not contemplated at this time, then reassessed at regular intervals.

The most obvious way of preventing glucocorticoid-induced osteoporosis is to stop corticosteroids. In most instances this is not possible for other reasons, but it is self-evident that the minimum effective dose should be utilized. In children the use of glucocorticoids is complicated by the effects of these agents on growth. Impairment of growth can be decreased by the alternate-day use of corticosteroids but appears to have little effect on osteoporosis (Chesney *et al.*, 1978). Children commonly fail to grow on daily doses as low as 0.5 mg/kg per day but may do so on 1 mg/kg per day each 48 hours.

Topical agents

Additional approaches to reducing the steroid burden are to use topical agents wherever possible. In the case of asthma many physicians now believe that inhaled corticosteroids can be used to control the disease in all but a very small minority of patients. Corticosteroids applied to the skin or inhaled are absorbed into the systemic circulation and have been shown to alter biochemical indices of skeletal metabolism (see Chapter 4). There is some evidence that growth in children is impaired on doses of beclomethasone of 400–1000 µg daily. Whether or not this is associated with significant bone loss is yet to be determined, but suggests that patients requiring long-term corticosteroids by these routes should also be monitored.

In some patients corticosteroid requirements can be decreased by the use of additional agents with less adverse effects on bone. Examples include the use of azathioprine in the context of transplantation and, more recently, the use of methotrexate in patients with chronic asthma or myasthenia. On the other hand, there is some evidence that cyclosporin might induce osteoporosis. There has also been considerable interest in the use of corticosteroid analogues which may have less adverse effects on skeletal metabolism.

DEFLAZACORT

Bone-sparing agents

Deflazacort is an oxazoline derivative of prednisone. A number of clinical studies have suggested that this agent may have fewer adverse effects than prednisone or prednisolone at doses with equivalent anti-inflammatory activity. Deflazacort has been found to have less marked short-term effects on intestinal calcium absorption. For 'equivalent' doses it also has less effect on biochemical markers of bone resorption such as the urinary excretion of calcium and hydroxyproline (Hahn *et al.*, 1980). Several studies have shown a slower rate of bone loss in patients given deflazacort compared with prednisone. One study has shown a similar effect utilizing histomorphometry as an end-point. In addition, it appears to have fewer adverse effects on the suppression of adrenal function and glucose tolerance (Table 9.1).

Dose equivalence

There is no doubt that deflazacort is an adequate anti-inflammatory agent. There are, however, two problems in the interpretation of the place of deflazacort in management. The first relates to the therapeutic equivalence of these agents with other corticosteroids. Many studies

Table 9.1 Mean serum cortisol (nmol/l ± SEM) before and 30 minutes and 1 hour after the intramuscular injection of 0.25 mg tetracosactrin in 18 patients established on long-term glucocorticoid therapy subsequently given deflazacort. (From Gray *et al.*, 1990)

	Before substitution	Three months after substitution
Baseline	145 ± 28	215 ± 43*
30 minutes	278 ± 48	408 ± 68†
60 minutes	277 ± 49	409 ± 59‡

Probability values denote the significance of differences before and after substitution with deflazacort.
* $P < 0.05$.
† $P < 0.01$.
‡ $P < 0.005$.

have suggested that 5 mg of prednisone or prednisolone is equivalent to 6 mg of deflazacort, but most clinical studies have made this a pretreatment assumption. The assumed dose equivalence may bias the assessment of therapeutic equivalence (Gray *et al.*, 1990). This can only be fully resolved with long-term studies making no such assumptions and utilizing a small tablet size.

Change in body mass

A second problem relates to the assessment of bone mineral density (BMD) since when deflazacort is substituted for prednisolone there is a marked change in body mass index (Gray *et al.*, 1990) which continues over at least 6 months and is likely to represent an increase in the ratio of lean body mass to fat tissue. This may affect absorptiometric measurements and overestimate the bone-sparing effects of deflazacort. Notwithstanding, decreased losses at the doses tested have been demonstrated utilizing histological techniques (LoCascio *et al.*, 1984) and from indirect indices of skeletal metabolism.

VITAMIN D AND DERIVATIVES

If hyperparathyroidism is a feature of glucocorticoid-induced osteoporosis (see Chapter 4) it might be expected that the stimulation of intestinal absorption with calcium would suppress the secretion of parathyroid hormone (PTH) and thereby decrease bone loss. Studies utilizing vitamin D derivatives have been on relatively few patients.

Suppression of hyperparathyroidism

Calcidiol together with calcium showed a marked increase in calcium absorption and decrease in PTH levels associated with a decreased bone resorption, as judged by osteoclast counts in biopsies. Forearm bone mineral content increased over the first year and thereafter the increment was less. Control subjects showed a non-significant decrease in BMD (Hahn *et al.*, 1979).

Many other studies have been undertaken utilizing dihydrotachysterol, the parent vitamin D, calcitriol and alfacalcidol. With the exception of one study utilizing calcitriol, rates of bone loss were attenuated in corticosteroid-treated patients. Indeed, the consistency of the observations is much greater than that in uncomplicated postmenopausal osteoporosis. There is some evidence that vitamin D is only effective when doses of prednisolone are less than 20 mg daily. The doses of vitamin D utilized have been 50 000 U three-times weekly for the parent vitamin, 40 µg daily for calcidiol and doses ranging from 0.4 to 1 µg daily for the 1-hydroxylated derivatives. As in the case of uncomplicated osteoporosis, care should be taken to avoid hypercalcaemia by appropriate monitoring.

CALCIUM

Most of the regimens described with vitamin D have also utilized calcium as a supplement. Several studies have looked at the effects of calcium supplements alone. As might be expected, the effects appear to be more modest, but their administration reduced the urinary excretion of hydroxyproline. Several studies have shown an attenuation of glucocorticoid-induced bone loss.

FLUORIDE

Several open and uncontrolled studies have shown that bone mass can be substantially increased with the use of sodium fluoride in patients treated with corticosteroids. Serial BMD measurements may increase markedly, but, as in the case of primary osteoporosis, the response is heterogeneous. In one small study the response in lumbar bone density in the first year to 20–30 mg of sodium fluoride ranged from 1 to 81% (Greenwald et al., 1992). In a well-controlled study, no change was noted in the appendicular skeleton (Rickers et al., 1982). Thus, the effects are similar to those observed in postmenopausal osteoporosis. No information is available concerning the effects on vertebral or hip fracture.

BISPHOSPHONATES AND CALCITONIN

Pamidronate, etidronate and clodronate have been tested in corticosteroid-induced osteoporosis. Intermittent cyclical etidronate given for 6 months with prednisone in postmenopausal women with temporal arteritis appears to prevent bone loss (Mulder & Snelder, 1992) at the lumbar spine. The dosage regimen is 400 mg daily for 2 out of every 13 weeks. No significant effects on BMD are reported at the femoral neck. The longest experience has been with pamidronate (150 mg daily) or clodronate utilizing a continuous regimen of 1200 mg daily. Changes in BMD occurred as predicted from experience in uncomplicated osteoporosis (Fig. 9.1).

In open studies parenteral calcitonin appears to inhibit steroid-induced bone loss over 1–2 years and similar results have been observed with nasally administered calcitonin.

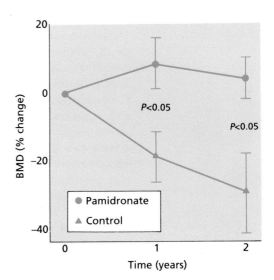

Fig. 9.1 Changes in vertebral bone mineral density (BMD) (mean ± SEM) in five patients treated with pamidronate and 11 control subjects. (From Reid *et al.*, 1988.)

ANABOLIC AND GONADAL STEROIDS

The glucocorticoids impair gonadal function and provide the rationale for the careful assessment of gonadal status both in men and in women before the menopause. There is some evidence that progestogens may compete at bone for glucocorticoid receptors, and appear to have beneficial effects on vertebral BMD. In addition, a retrospective study suggests that hormone replacement therapy (HRT) prevents bone loss for at least 1 year (Fig. 9.2). As might be expected, bone tissue in corticosteroid-treated patients also appears to be sensitive to the anabolic steroids.

A place for HRT

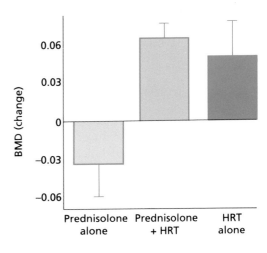

Fig. 9.2 Changes in bone mineral density (BMD) of the lumbar spine (mean ± SEM) over 1 year in postmenopausal or amenorrhoeic women taking prednisolone, hormone replacement therapy (HRT) or the combination. (From Lukert *et al.*, 1992.)

The pattern of glucocorticoid-induced osteoporosis in children is similar to that in adults. However, if steroids can be stopped before closure of the vertebral epiphyses then deformities may regress. There is only limited experience of the use of any bone-active agents in children. Some studies have suggested that the use of deflazacort may permit more normal growth. Since corticosteroids suppress growth hormone secretion there is some interest in its use, but early experience was disappointing. More recently, growth rates have been increased with recombinant human growth hormone. There is limited experience of the use of bisphosphonates in children. A small open but controlled study used clodronate 1200 mg daily for 1 year (Lepore et al., 1991). They observed an increase in vertebral mineral density of 7% judged by quantitative computerized tomography, whereas in untreated patients bone loss continued. The favourable experience of pamidronate in adults (see Fig. 9.1) also suggests that the bisphosphonates have an important role in the management of children.

Avascular necrosis gives rise most commonly to pain, but there is no proven medical treatment. Pain may resolve in time but recurs if there is collapse at the articular surface. At the hip it is usually treated by arthroplasty.

Hyperparathyroidism of the elderly

Low values for calcidiol are commonly found in the elderly, particularly those confined to institutional care. Whether or not this represents osteomalacia is another question but poor nutrition of vitamin D is one of several mechanisms for the induction of secondary hyperparathyroidism. Irrespective of the cause of hyperparathyroidism there is a case for screening the elderly for secondary hyperparathyroidism and to treat the disorder with vitamin D. A PTH value above normal using an intact assay or a calcidiol value of less than 20 nmol/l are appropriate intervention thresholds.

The active analogues of vitamin D (alfacalcidol, calcitriol and dihydrotachysterol; see Chapter 8) are inappropriate for prevention. They are certainly effective in treating privational vitamin D deficiency but their therapeutic window is narrow, so that toxicity is a problem. A more rational approach is the use of vitamin D_2 or vitamin D_3, which can be given alone or with calcium and other supplements where other nutritional deficits are suspected. In some countries combined formulations of calcium and vitamin D are available and are useful in the elderly where multiple tablet types increase the risk of non-compliance or toxicity. It is important, however, to check that the dose of vitamin D and calcium is appropriate.

Appropriate amounts of vitamin D are approximately 400 IU daily. Some believe that the requirements are greater in the elderly and for this reason give 800 IU daily. These doses may be preferable in patients taking phenytoin or barbiturates, but larger amounts may cause toxicity with time. Doses in the range of 10 000 to 50 000 IU daily, twice weekly or weekly are dangerous and should not be used. In patients who are unlikely to be compliant, intermittent intramuscular injection may be used. Annual injections of 150 000 or 300 000 IU can be given in the autumn and levels of calcidiol remain increased throughout the year.

Effects on fracture

The use of physiologically appropriate doses of vitamin D leads to the suppression of PTH and a decrease in bone loss. Two recently controlled prospective studies have shown a decrease in fracture rates in elderly individuals. The first (Chapuy *et al.*, 1992) was a double-blind prospective study in patients from a nursing home environment given placebo or a combination of calcium and vitamin D. This showed a significant decrease both in hip fractures and other fragility fractures over an 18-month period (see Chapter 7). The second study (Heikinheimo *et al.*, 1992) was partly based in the community and partly drawn from nursing homes. In this study an intramuscular injection of 150 000–300 000 IU was given annually to individuals aged 75 years or more. Treatment resulted in a significant decrease in fracture frequency (Table 9.2). The number of fractures at each site is insufficient to address site-specific effects, but the regimen did not appear to protect against vertebral fracture. The effects of vitamin D in the non-institutionalized elderly are less certain. Recent studies suggest that vitamin D has little effect on hip fracture rates in the general population where calcium nutrition is adequate (P. Lips, personal communication 1994). Effects may be confined, therefore, to the frail and those in institutionalized care.

Risks low

The risks of low-dose vitamin D supplementation are very low (Lips *et al.*, 1988) in the absence of sarcoidosis and idiopathic hyper-

Table 9.2 Effects of intramuscular vitamin D 150 000–300 000 IU annually on fractures in men and women aged 75 years or more at the sites shown. (Data from Heikinheimo *et al.*, 1992)

Site of fracture	Vitamin D (*n* = 341) Number (%)	Controls (*n* = 458) Number (%)
Vertebrae	8 (2.3)	6 (1.3)
Ribs and sternum	3 (0.9)	12 (2.6)
Pelvis	2 (0.6)	4 (0.9)
Humerus	3 (0.9)	11 (2.4)
Forearm	5 (1.5)	14 (3.1)
Femoral neck	25 (7.3)	43 (9.4)
All these sites	46 (13.5)	90 (19.7*)
These and other sites	56 (16.4)	100 (21.8*)

* Significantly different from controls.

calciuria. Although vitamin D status may also be improved by sunshine exposure and ultraviolet irradiation, the radiation required is higher in the elderly than in young adults (Holick, 1990). In addition, excessive sunshine exposure in the elderly increases the frequency of skin cancer.

Immobilization and fracture

Immobilization-induced bone loss, hypercalciuria and hypercalcaemia have all been effectively treated with clodronate, alendronate and the calcitonins. In the case of calcitonin, bone loss due to enforced bed rest was prevented over a 17-week period. Etidronate (900 mg daily) has also been shown in experimental subjects to attenuate bone loss due to bed rest but the effects were incomplete despite an exercise regimen.

The bisphosphonate clodronate has also been used in the immobilization associated with paraplegia and has been shown to decrease osteoclast numbers and prevent bone loss (Table 9.3). The same group has also studied the effects of calcitonin 100 IU 3 times weekly for 3 months and etidronate 20 mg/kg for 8 weeks and 10 mg/kg thereafter in patients with paraplegia. In contrast to the effects of clodronate, urinary calcium excretion did not decrease. In the case of etidronate this may well have been due to the high doses used which impaired the mineralization of bone. The lack of effect of calcitonin is not explained, particularly since in these studies bone appeared to be preserved at biopsy.

The bone loss that occurs in the distal segment after fracture can be substantial and most evidence suggests that this is at best only partially recoverable in adults (see Chapter 4). A recent open but randomized study has shown a partial effect of porcine calcitonin 10 Medical Research Council units given on alternate days (Ulivieri et al., 1994). The incomplete effects may be because relatively low doses of calcitonin were used.

Table 9.3 Effect of clodronate or placebo on bone mineral content (g/cm) of the distal tibia (mean ± SEM) in patients with spinal cord injury. (From Minaire et al., 1987)

	Before treatment	At 3 months	At 6 months
Placebo	1.99 ± 0.01	1.87 ± 0.02	1.85 ± 0.05
Clodronate			
400 mg daily	2.00 ± 0.04	1.92 ± 0.03	2.02 ± 0.06*
1600 mg daily	1.98 ± 0.05	1.93 ± 0.04	1.97 ± 0.05*

* Significantly different (P< 0.05) from placebo-treated patients.

Algodystrophy

A wide variety of treatments have been proposed for the treatment of algodystrophy (Table 9A). With a few exceptions, their role is uncertain. The major problem in the assessment of treatment is that the disorder tends to resolve spontaneously so that controlled trials of treatment are required. In addition, improvement may be very rapid indeed, and occasionally cases are seen where symptoms, present for many weeks beforehand, have disappeared overnight.

Spontaneous recovery

LOCAL TREATMENT

Physiotherapy is often the initial treatment of choice, either alone or in combination with other treatments. It is the general belief that early mobilization of an injured extremity prevents the development of algodystrophy. Although this sounds plausible it has never been tested and indeed may aggravate pain, swelling and stiffness. Physiotherapy encouraging the maintenance of movement is nevertheless appropriate, but should be tailored to the degree of pain and limitation of movement. For this reason most treatments have utilized physiotherapy as an adjunct to other specific treatments which affect pain.

During the past decade several reports of favourable results have been obtained with different kinds of transcutaneous nerve stimulators. There is some evidence that they may alter sympathetic tone, and there are anecdotal reports of its value in algodystrophy, particularly in children. A widely used treatment is sympathetic blockade, achieved either by regional sympathetic block or surgical sympathectomy. Alternatively, intravenous infusions of reserpine or guanethidine have been used which effectively produce a transient chemical sympathectomy. In a large series of patients, Steinbrocker *et al.* (1948) observed remissions in approximately 50% of patients after

Sympathectomy

Table 9A   Treatments used in algodystrophy

Conservative
Physiotherapy
Transcutaneous nerve stimulation
Miscellaneous, e.g., peripheral nerve stimulation, electro-acupuncture
Sympathetic interruption
Regional sympathetic blockade
Surgical sympathectomy
Cervical sympathectomy
Drug treatment
Corticosteroids
β-blockers
Calcitonin
Miscellaneous, e.g., griseofulvin, nifedipine, α-blockers

sympathetic blockade and this response rate was better than with the use of corticosteroids.

Surgical sympathectomy may be contemplated in patients with algodystrophy who have attained partial relief from regional sympathetic blockade but in whom relapse has occurred despite several treatments. Several large series have shown remission rates which average 84%. The follow-up in these series has ranged from 6 months to 17 years.

SYSTEMIC DRUG TREATMENT

Corticosteroids

Systemic corticosteroids have been widely used since the 1950s. Their effectiveness is, however, still relatively unproven. Several large but uncontrolled studies have been undertaken with high remission rates. In one of the few randomized controlled studies prednisolone 30 mg/day was compared to placebo given for up to 12 weeks. They observed that in all 13 patients treated with prednisolone the pretreatment score improved by 75%, whereas only 20% of patients who received placebo experienced relief (Christensen *et al.*, 1982). An alternative route for delivery of steroids is to combine methylprednisolone with regional blocks.

Many other drug treatments have been utilized, including griseofulvin, nifedipine, α-blockers and propranolol. These studies have all suffered from a lack of appropriate controls. The most widely utilized agent is calcitonin and there are many reports of its efficacy, particularly in the French literature. Several controlled trials have been

Calcitonin

undertaken using injected salmon calcitonin. In one (Doury *et al.*, 1981), 100 IU was given for 4 weeks in 28 patients with algodystrophy of the lower limbs. At 14 days there was an appreciable improvement in pain in 64% of those receiving calcitonin compared with a 25% response in the placebo group. At 28 days both groups had improved such that there was no longer any significant difference in their pain, suggesting that calcitonin accelerated the rate of response.

Neoplastic bone disease

Osteoporosis is a conspicuous feature of many neoplasms, but the archetype is myelomatosis where general rarefaction of bone is commonly observed. For this reason a great deal of attention has been directed to the use of bone-active agents in this disorder. Fluoride has been tested extensively and shown to increase bone mass. How-

Fluoride

ever, a double-blind randomized study of patients with myeloma showed a similar incidence of vertebral fracture between fluoride-treated patients (25 or 200 mg daily of sodium fluoride) and placebo (Harley *et al.*, 1972).

Since the major mechanism for skeletal resorption in neoplastic bone disease is due to the activation of osteoclasts, there has been a great deal of interest in the use of specific inhibitors of bone resorption such as the calcitonins and the bisphosphonates. Both classes of compounds have been successful in the acute management of hypercalcaemia, though the effects of calcitonin are less complete than the second generation bisphosphonates. Other inhibitors of bone resorption tested include mithramycin, gallium and non-steroidal anti-inflammatory agents, but they have been found either to be ineffective or their use limited by toxicity.

Calcitonin is an effective inhibitor of bone resorption in the context of the hypercalcaemia due to malignancy. Its effects are incomplete and with continued treatment relapse occurs which can be extended with the addition of glucocorticoids. Longer term experience either in the management of bone pain or to inhibit osteolysis, have given variable results. Several studies have shown beneficial short-term effects of calcitonin on bone pain or bone resorption but incomplete long-term effects are observed.

By far the most promising agents for osteolytic bone disease are the bisphosphonates. Etidronate has been tested in myelomatosis in a prospective double-blind study where the active wing received etidronate 5 mg daily. The study showed progressive height loss in both wings and there was no effect on bone pain, hypercalcaemia or pathological fractures (Belch *et al.*, 1991). In contrast, both clodronate and pamidronate are more suitable agents for the long-term control of osteolysis. Acute treatment with the use of oral (1600–3200 mg daily) or intravenous (600 mg) clodronate have shown a significant decrease of bone pain in normocalcaemic patients. Continued treatment is associated with a suppression of osteoclast-mediated bone resorption. Several studies have now shown that a sustained decrease in bone resorption occurs with long-term treatment with clodronate and is associated with a reduction in bone pain and a decrease in the extension as well as formation of new metastases in breast cancer (Table 9.4). A larger double-blind study showed a significant decrease

in the incidence of hypercalcaemia and vertebral fractures in women with skeletal relapse (Table 9.5). Similar effects of clodronate have

Table 9.4 Incidence of complications in 34 patients with breast cancer and skeletal metastases given clodronate or placebo for 1 year and followed for a further year. (From Elomaa *et al.*, 1987)

	Clodronate			Placebo		
	1 year	2 years	Total	1 year	2 years	Total
New bone metastases	3	11	14	11	9	20
Skeletal fractures	1	1	2	4	9	13
Episodes of hypercalcaemia	1	1	2	4	3	7
Survival	4	11	11	9	4	3

Table 9.5 Fracture rates (events/100 patient years) in women with breast cancer given continuous clodronate (1600 mg daily) or placebo. (From Paterson *et al.*, 1993)

	Clodronate (n = 85)	Placebo (n = 88)	P<
Non-vertebral fractures	32	40	–
Vertebral fractures	84	124	0.02
Vertebral deformity score	168	252	0.001

been noted in myelomatosis (Lahtinen *et al.*, 1992). As might be expected of an agent which has no intrinsic chemotherapeutic activity, survival is unaffected. Most dosage regimens have utilized between 1600 and 2400 mg daily on a continuous basis, which are higher than those generally used in osteoporosis. The incidence of side effects has been no different, however, between placebo and test wings.

Fewer studies of pamidronate are available but results are similar. It has been shown to reduce skeletal-related events in patients with bone metastases from breast cancer. Subsequent analyses have shown lesser effects (van Holten-Verzantvoort *et al.*, 1993). Gastrointestinal toxicity led to 25% of the patients withdrawing from the study at an early stage. Although reduction of the dose from 600 to 300 mg daily reduced this, it may have accounted for the attenuation of effect. As in the case of clodronate, the doses of pamidronate used are substantially greater than those used in the management of osteoporosis.

Improved quality of life

Survival of patients with myelomatosis or with skeletal involvement due to breast cancer has not improved substantially over the past 10 or 15 years. Against this background the ability of the bisphosphonates to improve the quality of life of affected patients is a substantial gain.

Miscellaneous disorders

Osteogenesis imperfecta

The management of osteogenesis imperfecta includes orthopaedic and supportive treatment together with counselling as appropriate. It is important to maintain mobility and muscle power. There is no proven medical intervention for the disorder, partly because of its rarity and its heterogeneous expression, which makes controlled trials difficult to undertake and evaluate. In adult women who present after the menopause, we commonly prescribe HRT, which certainly can prevent postmenopausal bone loss in these patients. Skeletal effects of the bisphosphonates are observed in osteogenesis imperfecta (Fig. 9.3), but whether this is of clinical significance is not known.

Gastrectomy and hepatobiliary diseases are associated with both osteoporosis and osteomalacia. It is important to exclude osteomalacia unless treatment with vitamin D is envisaged. In the absence of

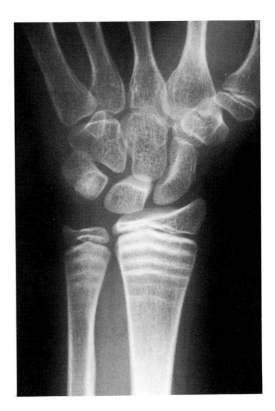

Fig. 9.3 Effect of intermittent pamidronate given every 3 months to a child of 12 years with osteogenesis imperfecta. Note the marked and persistent sclerosis at the sites of growth. (From Devogelaer *et al.*, 1987.)

vitamin D deficiency, there is little evidence for its efficacy. Treatment with pharmacological doses of calcium (1000 mg daily) delay bone loss at the metacarpal in biliary cirrhosis and similar responses have been shown in patients concurrently taking corticosteroids for chronic active hepatitis.

Many of the rarer secondary causes of osteoporosis have been treated on an *ad hoc* basis, but have clearly shown drug-induced responses which can be attributable to the agent. Their long-term effects are of course not known. Examples include the increased bone resorption due to mastocytosis, eosinophilic granuloma, congenital erythropoietic porphyria and Gaucher's disease. In many instances, these disorders have responded to the bisphosphonates.

References

Belch AR, Bergsagel DE, Wilson K *et al.* (1991) Effect of daily etidronate on the osteolysis of multiple myeloma. *J Clin Oncol*; **9**: 1397–1402.

Chapuy MC, Arlot ME, Dubneuf F *et al.* (1992) Vitamin D₃ and calcium to prevent hip fractures in elderly women. *N Engl J Med*; **327**: 1637–1642.

Chesney RW, Mazess RB, Rose P, Jax DK (1978) Effect of prednisone on growth and bone mineral content in childhood glomerular disease. *Am J Dis Child*; **132**: 768–772.

Christensen K, Jensen EM, Noer I (1982) The reflex dystrophy syndrome response to treatment with systemic steroids. *Acta Chir Scand*; **148**: 653–655.

Devogelaer JP, Malghem J, Maldague B, Nagant de Deuxchaisnes C (1987) Radiological manifestations of bisphosphonate treatment with APD in a child suffering from osteogenesis imperfecta. *Skeletal Radiol*; **16**: 360–363.

Doury P, Dirheimer Y, Pattin S (1981) *Algodystrophy: Diagnosis and Therapy of a Frequent Disease of the Locomotor Apparatus.* Springer-Verlag, Berlin.

Elomaa I, Blomqvist C, Porkka L *et al.* (1987) Treatment of skeletal disease in breast cancer. A controlled clodronate trial. *Bone*; **8** (suppl.): 53–56.

Gray RES, Harrington C, Coulton L *et al.* (1990) Long-term treatment of chronic inflammatory disorders with deflazacort. *J Orthop Rheumatol*; **3**: 15–27.

Greenwald M, Brandli D, Spector S *et al.* (1992) Corticosteroid-induced osteoporosis: effects of a treatment with slow-release sodium fluoride. *Osteoporosis Int*; **2**: 303–304.

Hahn TJ, Halstead LR, Teitelbaum SL, Hahn BH (1979) Altered mineral metabolism in glucocorticoid-induced osteopenia. Effect of 25-hydroxyvitamin D administration. *J Clin Invest*; **64**: 655–665.

Hahn TJ, Halstead LR, Strates B *et al.* (1980) Comparison of subacute effects of oxazacort and prednisone on mineral metabolism in man. *Cacif Tissue Int*; **31**: 109–115.

Harley JB, Schilling A, Glidewell O (1972) Ineffectiveness of fluoride therapy in multiple myeloma. *N Engl J Med*; **286**: 1283–1288.

Heikinheimo RJ, Inkovaara JA, Harju EJ *et al.* (1992) Annual injection of vitamin D and fractures of aged bones. *Calcif Tissue Int*; **51**: 105–110.

Holick MF (1990) Vitamin D and the skin: photobiology, physiology, and therapeutic efficacy for psoriasis. In Heersche JMM, Kanis JA (eds). *Bone and Mineral Research Annual 7*, pp. 313–366. Elsevier, Amsterdam.

Lahtinen R, Laakso M, Palva I *et al.* (1992) Randomized placebo-controlled multicentre trial of clodronate in multiple myeloma. *Lancet*; **340**: 1049–1052.

Lepore L, Pennesi M, Barbi E, Pozzi R (1991) Treatment and prevention of osteoporosis in juvenile chronic arthritis with disodium clodronate. *Clin Exp Rheumatol*; **9** (suppl. 6): 33–35.

Lips P, Wiersinga A, van Ginkel FC *et al.* (1988) The effect of vitamin D supplementation on vitamin D status and parathyroid function in elderly subjects. *J Clin Endocrinol Metab*; **67**: 644–650.

LoCascio V, Bonucci E, Imbimbo B *et al.* (1984) Bone loss after glucocorticoid therapy. *Calcif Tissue Int*; **36**: 435–438.

Lukert BP, Johnson BE, Robinson RG (1992) Estrogen and progesterone replacement therapy reduces glucocorticoid-induced bone loss. *J Bone Miner Res*; **7**: 1063–1069.

Minaire P, Depassio J, Berard E *et al.* (1987) Effects of clodronate on immobilization bone loss. *Bone*; **8**: 563–568.

Mulder H, Snelder HAA (1992) Effect of cyclical etidronate regimen on prophylaxis of bone loss of glucocorticoid therapy in postmenopausal women. *Bone Miner*; **17** (suppl. 1): A955.

Paterson AHG, Powles TJ, Kanis JA *et al.* (1993) Oral clodronate decreases skeletal morbidity in patients with bone metastases for breast cancer. A double blind controlled trial. *J Clin Oncol*; **11**: 59–69.

Reid IR, Heap SW, King AR, Ibbertson HK (1988) Two-year follow-up of bisphosphonate (APD) treatment in steroid osteoporosis. *Lancet*; **ii**: 1144.

Rickers H, Deding A, Christiansen C *et al.* (1982) Corticosteroid-induced osteopenia and vitamin D metabolism. Effect of vitamin D_2, calcium phosphate and sodium fluoride administration. *Clin Endocr*; **16**: 409–415.

Steinbrocker O, Spitzer N, Freidman HH (1948) The shoulder–hand syndrome in reflex dystrophy of the upper extremity. *Ann Intern Med*; **29**: 22–52.

Ulivieri FM, Bossi E, Ronzani C *et al.* (1994) Prevention of bone loss with calcitonin in fractured leg. *Bone*; in press.

van Holten-Verzantvoort ATM, Kroon HM *et al.* (1993) Palliative pamidronate treatment in patients with bone metastases from breast cancer. *J Clin Oncol*; **11**: 491–498.

Index